STRESS FREE YOU!

Discover how to turn off stress with the flick of a switch

Matt Rush & Rich Taylor

Rhema Communications Group
Tampa, Florida

ISBN: 9798634661988

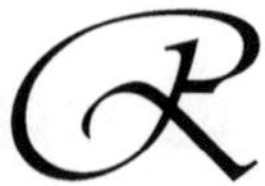

DEDICATION

This book is a montage of true, entertaining, enlightening and often touching illustrations to encourage you on your journey to a stress-free life.

Whether you are an eight-year-old with parents yelling in the next room or the CEO of the world's large organization, we wrote this book as an easy to read guide for you. While we are not scientists or doctors, we are two observant dudes who spent decades learning how to turn off the stress switches in our lives. Now, it is our passion and calling to pass the stress-free life along to everyone.

Stress Free You is dedicated to all of you who have let stress paint you into a corner. We hope you find your freedom.

Check out the Stress Free You podcast that can be found wherever you get your podcasts.

StressFreeYou.net

CONTENTS

ACKNOWLEDGMENTS

This book would not be possible without our editor, Cynthia Beal.

I want to thank my wonderful wife Donna who stood with me throughout this entire process. I could not have done it without you. –Rich

Finally, there is one beautiful soul who deserves a specific note of appreciation. She not only contributed to part of this book, but she also is a co-host on our weekly podcast. Katy Rush, you truly make us better in every way. –Matt

INTRODUCTION

Twenty-three years ago, I was walking out of my office when I asked myself this question, "Why can't people who start any form of positive life change stay with it? Why do people fail at staying on diets, workout regimes, budgets, etc.?" At the time, I was deeply immersed in working in the motivational seminar business. Throughout my career, I witnessed over 11 million people come through our events. Without fail, they got fired up with enthusiasm! A few might have even gotten fired with enthusiasm. These attendees were taught by some of the most successful people in the world; like former US Presidents, world leaders, sports legends, Hollywood actors, business leaders, etc. The knowledge that was imparted by these legendary leaders was life-changing and priceless. But the question that has plagued me since then is, "How many of those 11 million people made positive life changes that lasted?"

They left every one of our events filled with such fantastic knowledge, but why didn't they change? Why didn't it last?

Then twenty-three years later, I received the answer in one word: stress.

The attendees of those events did not lack information, inspiration, or even perspiration. Stress stopped them in their tracks, just like it has so many of us.

We have designed this book to be as stress-less as possible. It is a soft read, not a hard sell. We chose soft pastel colors for the cover. We seldom mention any diseases by name to keep you from being even more stressed. Our goal is not to scare you into a behavior change but to enlighten you so you can make an informed decision about your life and truly wake up each day with hope.

Rich Taylor, Co-Author

Do you remember when Walmart had a greeter stationed at the door to welcome you to their store? As you walked in, they would typically say, “Welcome to Walmart. We hope you have a great day.” It was like having a grandparent welcome you into the store. I loved the greeters.

My absolute favorite was a special needs girl named Tabby. She always wore a bow on top of her head that would make Minnie Mouse jealous. Whenever Tabby was on duty, as soon as the automatic doors opened, she would enthusiastically say in the most distinctive voice, “Weeeeellllllcome to Waaaaaaaaalllllllllllll-Mart! How ya doin there, buddy? I hope you have a gggggrrreat day!” She was THE BEST. I loved Tabby.

At that time in my life, I was beginning my career as an inspirational and motivational speaker. Aspiring to be more positive than anyone else, I made it a game to greet the greeter with a greeting before they could greet me. Upon entering the store, with Tabby stationed at her post, I beat her to the punch by saying, “WELL HELLO TABBY! How are YOU doing today?”

Her response back still resonates in my ears. She said, “OPTIMISTICALLY FANTASTIC!” I laughed out loud! I said, “Well, you can’t get much better than that; can you Tabby?”
She said, “Not a chance, Buddy!”

Shouldn’t we all be able to live a life with that kind of optimism, encouragement, and hope?

We KNOW that you can! We also know that the first step is to rid yourself of the stress that has weighed you down and kept you from it. *Stress Free You* can help you live a life that really is "optimistically fantastic."

Matt Rush, Co-Author

Maybe you've heard the parable about a man who was walking down the road and fell into a bottomless, dark, steep hole. He could not figure out how to get out of the hole. A doctor walked by, and he yelled up from the hole, "Hey, can you help me? I've fallen into this hole and cannot get out!"

The doctor wrote a prescription, threw it into the hole, and walked on. Then a preacher walked by, and the man yelled from the hole, "Hey, can you help me? I've fallen into this hole and cannot get out!" The preacher wrote scripture on a piece of paper, threw it into the hole, and walked on by. Then the man saw a friend walking by, and he yelled up to the friend, "Hey, Joe! Can you help me? I've fallen into this hole and cannot get out!" Joe jumped down in the hole beside his friend.

The man said, "Are you crazy? Now we're both in the hole!"

Joe smiled and said to his friend, "Yes, but I've been here before, and I know the way out!"

We know the way out! Welcome to Stress Free You!!!

CHAPTER ONE
HOW TO SUCCESSFULLY HANDLE STRESS

You can't. You have to switch it off.

CHAPTER TWO

THAT'S IT?

Caution: Heavy Chapter Ahead

As you begin this journey to the "stress-free you," most of what you will experience will be lighthearted, positive thoughts and suggestions; however, this first chapter is heavier than most. We want to get this out of the way so the rest of the journey will be smooth sailing to the best version of you that you could ever imagine!

One day you find yourself lying in bed, staring at the ceiling of your hospital room. As the clock on the wall ticks away the seconds to minutes to hours, your entire life passes before your eyes.

You have only hours of life left on this side of eternity. You can hear the mumbled sounds of your loved ones talking about stepping out of the room, but they hesitate in fear of missing your passing. You listen to them saying that "it won't be long and that you lived a good life." You are too weak to talk, and your organs are beginning to shut down one by one.

You think to yourself, "What good did I do in this life? What legacy am I leaving?" It all seems like nothing but a blur now, as you see your life fast-forwarding before your eyes.

From early childhood, it was constant stress: hurry up, do this and hurry up, do that. Then off to school where you hurried from one class to another, all marked by alarm bells. After school was filled with extracurricular activities, chores, homework, rinse, and repeat. Until the day came, and you made it through high school.

Then came the summer jobs, the heavy college course load so you could graduate early and start your adult life.

After college, you worked endless hours to build a career and make money while climbing the corporate ladder. Countless late nights at the office and all those extended business trips, until after many years, you finally reach the top of your field. You achieved your career success! Then it was time to retire.

Retirement seemed to consist of getting up early to beat the traffic to the golf course, play a round of 18 holes in record time. You count how long each traffic light is and are annoyed when you get a red light. You hurry to the dinner restaurant to get the early bird special. Whew!!

As you lie there, about to pass into eternity, you realize that almost every stinking day of your life has been a stressed-out combination of go, go, go, hurry, hurry, hurry, STRESS, STRESS, STRESS! You can scarcely imagine the millions, if not billions, of people who have followed this same path, only to have regrets at the end of their lives, knowing that they have spent their entire life chasing their tails to no avail.

How many people have sacrificed for “things” and money? In the end, those sacrifices might get you a nicer hospital room, but there has never been a “U-Haul” hooked to the back of a hearse. Never let the urgent replace the important.

You only have one life to live, so live it well! STRESS FREE YOU is THE tool to help you live your true life: one that is not ruled by stress, a life that is blessed and not stressed! Welcome to the journey to the new you, we love you.

CHAPTER THREE
THE STRESS-FREE LIFESTYLE

In a perfect world, you would have no problems.
In a perfect world, you would get along with everyone.
In a perfect world, you would weigh the exact pounds you would want to weigh, have as much money as you want to have, and do everything you want to do.
In a perfect world, you would never have any challenges.
In a perfect world, there would be no stress.

Unfortunately, you do not live in a perfect world. You live far, far from it. Every day it feels like you are bombarded with this stress or that stress or old stress or new stress.

If you are like the majority of people in the world, then you know what it is like to be stressed. If you are stressed, then you require relief. Stress Free You is the recipe you have been longing for to give you the lifestyle that you were designed to live. Stress is best described as being in a dangerous situation you have no control over. The obvious question to ask then, is it even possible to live stress-free in a stressed-out world? The answer is YES!

The world is full of experts and gurus who have compiled countless "How To" programs. They get rich selling you the solution to your problems. They arm you with every defense to lead you to the path of achieving the goal that you cannot achieve on your own. Yet with every fat burning, self-help, debt relief, money making program that is bought, 94% of them fail. Just because you live in "The Information Age" does not mean that Dr. Google and every other self-proclaimed Doctor of Information can solve all your problems. They keep coming out with new diets and self-help programs, which is proof that everything before didn't work.

What then is the one thing that everyone overlooks that causes such dismal performance? The answer is ***STRESS!***

You can have all the motivation to start, all the desire to begin again, and all the willpower to continue, but whenever that first stress event hits you, you go right back to your old "go-to" ways. Almost every time, you turn to some form of self-indulgence that you hope will fill the hole, ease the pain, and numb the stress. Bam! You have been derailed yet again. And once again, you are left feeling guilty and defeated.

Most people who go on a food diet have a 94% failure rate. That means that diets only have a dismal 6% chance of seeing any success. Ask yourself, how many diets or improvement programs have you tried? How many have worked? Here is some news that may shock you; most of them will work. Yes, despite the pathetic failure rate of these programs, most of them work. But ONLY IF YOU FOLLOW THEM.

So, what is the common denominator destroying almost every self-improvement program? ***STRESS!*** Stress will blow away even the most potent motivation and willpower in seconds. It is like putting an ice cube on the road at noon in Death Valley in the summer, where the surface temperature can reach as high as 200 degrees Fahrenheit.

Stress is the one thing most people who start a food diet or any positive life change never account for, and yet it is by far the most destructive force to any of them. We have been trained that, in times of stress, we are to resort to hedonistic pleasures. [Hedonist: Someone who is solely focused on the pursuit of self-gratification and what gives them pleasure.]

Have you ever noticed when you feel stressed, you seldom feel like eating a bowl of raw broccoli? No, we all want some instant gratification. It usually involves something sweet, carbs, or fat. This is because we are genetically engineered to crave those foods when we are stressed. In a stressed state, the body says, give me quick energy, because a saber-tooth tiger is chasing me, and I need to escape.

The training of society and advertising has destroyed our natural response and manipulated our "Go-To" for their profit.

Everyone has a "Go-To." Your "Go-To" is what you crave or do in times of stress. As children, you were rewarded with food when you performed well. "Great job, Mikey, you get a cookie." Or your mom says, "I know you had a tough day at school. I will make your favorite comfort food." There were always advertisements of restaurants continually telling you that you "need a break today." Food treats are great rewards for your pets, but they were never meant for human consumption.

Some people have healthy "Go-Tos." When stressed, you may "Go-To" clean the house, weed the garden, or "Go-To" the gym and work out or even help someone in need. You can't get much better "Go-To" than helping someone, but it is still not enough. The reason is, you are still allowing stress to affect you, and now you are trying to cover it up.

You can even have a fantastic loving family, a great job with a ton of money in the bank, your retirement fully funded, and the ability to take a nice vacation whenever you like. Having stress in your life will almost always keep you from enjoying all that life has to offer.

Note: stress is a significant factor in lowering people's immune systems, making them susceptible to disease. This is one of the few times we will ever mention anything about sickness. Most diet books spend chapters extolling the virtues of their diet in preventing this disease or the other. Just the mention of illness is stressful, so that is why we will not mention it any further.

To have any success in any area of your life, you must learn to live without stress. It truly is possible and will be revealed to you in more detail throughout this book. However, this book is not about how to manage stress but about how to live stress-free. Just like water rolling off a duck's back, stress will not affect you as it did before *Stress Free You.* Stress may have beaten you then, but NOT ANYMORE!

One of the significant benefits of *Stress Free You* is that it is not about doing more but doing less and getting amazing results. The mistake most people make is they attempt to do some type of stress relief to lower their stress levels rather than learning how to turn off the stress switches that continually increase their stress. It is like trying to drain your cell phone battery while it is still plugged into the power.

Stress Switches are the "things" that we have allowed to usher stress into our lives. There are hundreds, if not thousands, of common stress switches; many of them are hidden in plain sight. *Stress Free You* has uncovered these stress switches, and it is our mission to help you identify these stress switches, understand how they have turned stress on in your life, and, most importantly, how you can turn them off and eliminate stress.

Throughout this book, you will be hearing from two of the most stress-free people you will ever meet, Rich Taylor and Matt Rush. After decades of living stressed-out lifestyles, they found a way to turn off the stress switches that were causing stress. They both practice what they preach and believe that it is their calling and passion to help you live a stress-free lifestyle.

A personal note from Rich:

It is not only possible to live a stress-free lifestyle in theory and on paper but also in reality. I have been doing it for years with amazing results. Yes, I have a family with two awesome adult children, and like all parents, I did experience the "growing up phase" they went through as part of any normal life. I have been the sole owner and employee of my graphic design firm that I work by myself. My business is very deadline orientated and full of pressure. It is not unusual for a client to email me at 10 AM with a project that they need for a meeting or webinar that is at 3 pm that day. That can be stressful if you let it.

I remember we had an executive from a local advertising agency come to my class, where I attended school at Ringling College of Art and Design. He wanted to know if any of us could design a project for him. One of the more gifted students in the class asked him when he needed it done by. His reply was, "I needed it yesterday!" That is when I realized that I was getting into a profession with a lot of potential high-pressure situations. I have been a graphic designer for over 40 years and have been in some intense deadlines and massive amounts of work. I remember one year I worked from seven AM to midnight, six days a week, for over eight months straight. When you are the only person in your company, there is no one else to turn to. I earned a lot of money, but was it worth the stress? I did not truly begin to live until I began to live stress-free.

No matter who you are, what you do, or where you live, you have been impacted by stress. The moment you make that choice to live stress free, is the moment you can begin to create the life you were born to have. Welcome to a journey of a stress-free life!

A personal note from Matt:

As I travel around the country, I am constantly asked if I ever have a bad day. The answer is, of course, I do, everyone does, but even in those days, there is something to be grateful for. Throughout the ups and downs of life, there have been moments when I felt defeated, but I never let stress win and have hopefully always chosen to be a positive influence. Just like one day when I was checking out at a store, I noticed the checker didn't seem to be in the best of moods. As a "motivational speaker and farm boy," I decided to attempt cheering her up. I approached the register and exuberantly said, "GOOD DAY MA'AM! How are YOU today?!?" She looked up and said, rather expressionless, "I'm good. How are you?" I proudly said, "I'm goodER!" She laughed! That is when I decided that my motto would become, "Life is good. Let's make it GOODER!" I'm proud to be the "Gooder Guy" and help you have a gooder life.

That is why, when Rich approached me with the concept for STRESS FREE YOU, I was immediately excited. His approach is accurate in that getting rid of stress will positively change your life. I believe that it is a gift he was given from God and a legitimate way to help you live the life you were born to live. I am honored to be a part of it and thrilled you are coming along for the ride.

The approach of *Stress Free You* is radically different from any other program you have ever seen or heard. The tips that we will share with you are groundbreaking, genuinely potent, occasionally controversial, and positively life-changing.

If you want to try again and succeed,
If you want to start again and win,
If you want to give it your all and wake up every morning with hope,

Stress Free You is for YOU!

YOU DESERVE TO LIVE STRESS FREE!

CHAPTER FOUR

MOTIVATION, WILLPOWER AND STRESS

Motivation is the spark that becomes a flame and gets everything started. Nothing would ever get accomplished without motivation. As important and influential as motivation is, it suffers from a very short life-span. It can fade from the scene rather quickly.

Undoubtedly, your motivation ignites your willpower. Willpower is like a lightbulb. Some people have one or two, and some have more: the more bulbs, the more willpower. If you have the willpower to do something long enough, it will turn into a "new" habit. The problem is that most people never make it to the "new" habit phase. The culprit is the one overlooked villain hidden in plain sight: Stress.

Even if you have great willpower — say, 14 lightbulbs in all, stress is like a lightning bolt that blows up all the bulbs, or willpower, in the blink of an eye. When you are stressed, your first reaction is to revert to your old habits. Stress is the big bully that almost always wins.

For example: If you want to go skydiving, there is specific training you MUST go through. The one thing expert trainers focus on is creating a "new" habit. You are repeatedly trained on how you should react if your main parachute fails to deploy. I cannot think of a more stressful situation than plummeting toward earth from 10,000 feet with a defective parachute. It is easy to see why someone would panic and forget everything that you were taught. That is why you are repetitively taught what to do if that severe stress happens to you. The experts train you on how to stay calm and deploy your reserve parachute. The training is repeated so many times; it becomes your "new" habit.

Regrettably, most people fail to address their stress before they start a significant life change, like starting an exercise program. They usually start because of being stressed about the condition of their bodies. They finally get tired of feeling out of shape and low on energy and decide to start jogging every day before work. That spark is motivation and ignites willpower.

The next day they rise extra early, put on their brand-new running shoes and stretchy pants, and go for a jog. A little sore, but they do it consecutively for the next three days. Each day their willpower gets stronger and stronger. By lightbulb five, I mean day five, they are on the way to a successful "new" habit of jogging every morning. Note: a university study shows that most new habits become automatic after 66 days of repetition.

However, then stress strikes, and they have a banger day at work. The boss yells and threatens the team, and they all feel stressed out. They go out after work commiserating and consoling each other. They arrive home later than usual, and the next morning decide to sleep in because sleeping in is their "Go-To." It is what they always did when feeling stressed. Their light bulbs just got obliterated by a lightning bolt of stress. They skip jogging for the next couple of days, and before they know it, they are back to their old ways.

Sound familiar? Have you ever been in those shoes?

That is why it is imperative to reduce your stress BEFORE starting any form of self-improvement.

Otherwise, you stand about a six percent chance at success. Stress almost always wins. It will eat your lunch and steal your cookies. If we all lived in a stress-free world, our lives would be vastly different.

The good news is that you really can live stress-free and then be able to succeed in multiple positive life changes. You just have to deal with stress first.

There are more than enough experts out there preaching excellent programs on how to succeed at almost anything. The one thing most of them do not account for is stress. Again, you need to address the stress to be a success. Just remember that the strength that is within you may not be a flame that can be seen by the world, it may just be a tiny, little spark that whispers, “There’s no need to stress. You can do this.”

As you continue with Stress Free You, you will start to see the levels of stress in your life fade away. Living stress-free in a stressed-out world is possible. Motivation is a spark that will become a flame, and we call it discipline. You can do it!

CHAPTER FIVE

WHAT IS STRESS AND ITS EFFECTS

Stress is pressure or tension exerted on you.
Stress, by definition, is our response to mental or physical danger.
Stress is the external force that weighs us down.
Stress is the internal parasite that gnaws at our core.
Stress is quickly becoming the number one disease of our century.

What controls your stress?

Everything that happens in your body, including stress, is controlled by your Central Nervous System. This complex nervous system regulates all of the processes in your body. Many of which work automatically without any conscious effort on your part. This system is broken down into three types of nerves.

1. Motor nerves, which help our brain command our muscles to move or not to move.

2. Sensory nerves, which help us to see, smell, taste, hear, and feel.

3. The Autonomic Nervous System controls the internal organs. It is divided into two parts: The Sympathetic and the Parasympathetic.

The **Sympathetic Nervous System** prepares our bodies for action. Our fearfully and wonderfully made bodies are designed to react to a threat by preparing our bodies for action with only three options: fight, flight, or freeze. All the organs involved in getting ready for a physical challenge or preparing for a retreat are activated through your Sympathetic Nervous System. For example, if you are on your morning jog and a mean dog starts chasing you, your body automatically switches into fight, flight, or freeze mode in response to the danger. You can either choose to fight the dog, escape by running away or freeze in place. However, your sympathetic nervous system can also be triggered by ordinary things we experience daily like, the ringing of a phone, your morning alarm, or simply being pulled in too many directions.

The **Parasympathetic Nervous System** is our rest, digest, and restore system and helps us produce a state of "peace" in the body. The parasympathetic is a much slower system that is responsible for the balance and maintenance of the body's systems. When this is activated, our heart slows, and our breathing calms down. When we don't need to "fight, flight or freeze," our body sends blood to our organs and skeletal muscles. We digest our food, repair our muscles, build strength, and our body is in a state of relaxation, which helps our body heal. It restores the body to a state of calm and allows us to relax, digest, and repair.

Overall, the two parts of the nervous system work together to ensure that your body responds appropriately to different situations.

However, as you are fully aware, you and your sympathetic nervous system are dealing with many stressful situations. These stressful situations can be caused by outside forces, like a looming work deadline, or internal forces like persistent worry about losing your job.

Regardless of the source, when you experience stress, your body dumps hormones into your bloodstream that trigger a variety of changes. Your heart may pound, you can become short of breath, your muscles tense, beads of sweat form on your head, your stomach aches, your mouth goes dry, your mind races. All these symptoms are triggered by stress. These hormones pull energy away from your vital organs and send them into your muscles to make you ready to fight, run, or freeze in place. Non-essential systems like digestion and immunity are given a much lower priority, while more energy is directed to your muscles and your heart rate. It dramatically increases your awareness and heart rate with an almost superhuman boost of energy. It is the reason that people can do extraordinary things when faced with significant stress, without even thinking about the reality of the situation.

At best, you were designed only to activate the fight, flight, or freeze response a few times in your lives. The normal state for your body is rest, digest and repair. That is the place where you are allowing your body to heal from the usual wear and tear of your daily routine. However, in today's world, there seems little time for rest and repair.

Our bodies can react to stressors that are not life-threatening, such as pressure at work, family issues, commuting with traffic, etc. Over time, the constant activation of our fight, flight, or freeze response can have serious emotional, mental, and physical ramifications.

Stress is by far the most dangerous thing people face with regards to their health. You can eat super healthy, get the proper amount of sleep and exercise, live in a clean home, and do everything exactly right, but if stress invades, your health will fade. If you are exposed to continued stress, it can overwhelm everything that you do well and leave you with a significantly suppressed immune system. That can open the door to a host of catastrophic problems.

A note from Rich:

In the late 1970s, my dad was in his early 50's and took a position running a local insurance office. The office was ranked 348th in the country. His task was to take a broken, unsuccessful business and turn it around. Because of his leadership, within two years, he raised it to 14th in the country. My dad has always been a hard worker, gave it his all at work, and the results showed.

Many times, I remember him coming home complaining about how very stressful his job was. He said that he felt like he was doing a job that a much younger man should do. Even though he did a fantastic job, there were still things outside of his control that brought increased stress. He would often complain that when his agents sold a policy and submitted the paperwork to the regional office for processing, they would be either slow to process it or lose the paperwork.

On one such occasion, one of my dad's top agents sold a substantial policy and submitted it for processing. The regional office lost the paperwork resulting in the customer becoming incredibly frustrated and canceling the order. This cost both the agent and my dad a hefty commission. Can you imagine how stressful it would have been to break this news to your best agent?

After two years at that stressful job, my dad started complaining of pain in his lungs. The doctor first thought it was pleurisy, which causes pain when breathing. After a couple of weeks of no improvement, they took a chest X-Ray that showed his lungs were full of cancer. He was admitted to Sloan Kettering in New York City and was told that without treatment, he had only a couple of weeks to live. They immediately did surgery on his lungs and also removed a lot of his lymph nodes. Post-surgery he went through several intense treatments of experimental chemotherapy followed by monthly outpatient chemo treatments.

This all happened in the 1970s, when there were a lot of experimental drug trials and testing. I will spare you the gruesome details of what he went through. However, my dad is a warrior, and he pushed himself to get better. I am grateful to say that my dad made it to the marvelous age of 94 years old before he passed. My dad has always been my hero.

Everything that my dad went through might not have happened had he not been exposed to his stressful job. At the very least, if he had known how to identify stress, he could have turned those switches off so his body could focus on healing itself.

Over and over, we are told that a little stress can be a good motivator. We even have people tell us that they work better under pressure. However, there is no safe level of stress. For example, which is better, having a giant black widow spider or a small black widow spider in your bed? We do not want EITHER! Stress (and spiders in your bed) are bad.

Stress is the number one driving factor to virtually every problem that you face. All difficulties are exponentially worsened by stress. If you do not turn off your stress switches, you will be turning on increased problems.

Beyond the effects that stress can have on your physical life, it can have detrimental effects on other aspects of your life as well.

"Remember, the issue is rarely the issue." –Matt Rush

That is to say, if someone you know overreacts negatively to a situation or they are challenging to work with over something insubstantial, you can be assured that something else is going on. Stress is bleeding from one area of their life into another.

You have probably heard it said that you should keep your personal life separate from your professional life and vice versa. However, is it even possible to separate the two? Absolutely not! Think about target practice with a bow and arrow. To hit the bullseye, the arrow has to be in alignment. Imagine the front of your arrow is your personal life, and the back of the arrow is your professional life. If you have stress at home, your work-life will be affected. If you have stress at work, your life at home will likewise be affected. However, when you can recognize stress and switch it off, you will be much more apt to hit your target.

Stress will affect every area of your life. We all know that it is true. We have all experienced it personally.
Stress is pressure or tension exerted on you.
Stress is the external forces that weigh us down.
Stress is the internal parasites that gnaw at our core.
Stress is our body's reaction to danger.
Avoid stress at all costs, or else it could cost you all you have.

That is why living stress free is so vitally important to your entire being.

Amazingly enough, no one has probably ever given you permission to turn off the stress that has been impacting every area of your life. We are not only giving you that permission, but we are going to help you make it happen.

You were designed to live a life filled with love, joy, peace of mind, and excellent health.

You are now on your path to a stress free you.

CHAPTER SIX
HOW TO AVOID THE PINBALL RALLY

"How are you today?" he asked. She said, "I'm good. You?" "Doing good," he said. To which she replied, "That's good."

For decades, that was the standard greeting between two people. Whether anyone was ever actually "Good," we may never know, but that was just how a typical greeting went.

Today, when asked the same rhetorical question, the almost universal reply is that you are, "Busy!" Whenever you meet someone and ask him or her how they are, they will robotically reply, they are busy. No matter if you ask a CEO, a stay-at-home mom, a blue-collar worker, a student or someone unemployed, the answer is almost always the same, "I am SO BUSY!" It has gotten to the point that it is worn like a badge of honor or an official job title. People are all running around, going here or there, being stressed out, and genuinely feeling guilty if they are not busy. People have become busy at being busy.

Seriously, how can everyone be so busy and still have zero downtime? If any amount of stress is harmful, then why have you allowed your schedule to become one of the most stressful parts of your day?

The reality is, you were not designed to be a human pinball bouncing here and there and everywhere. It is not sustainable. It is not realistic. It is a major Stress Switch that you have been convinced cannot be turned off. Being busy is bad. It is really, really bad.

BUSY stands for Being Under Stress' Yoke.

The weight of the yoke will eventually cause you to stumble and fall. It is not physically, emotionally, or mentally possible to be busy 24 hours per day, seven days a week. You were not made to be that way. More importantly, it is okay to accept that. We were designed to only be active during daylight hours. That was the only time our ancestors could work. Today, we have been programmed by our stressed-out society to stay ON all the time. Because of technology, we are now ON even when we are supposed to be OFF.

I know some "super-achievers" brag about how little they sleep and how hard they work. That typically makes the rest of us feel less than successful if we are not living up to that same work ethic. I always heard that people who brag about how hard they work would lie about other things as well. Yet we have fallen into the trap of being busy to the point that it makes us feel important if we have at least ten balls in the air at the same time. When you look at the average person's resume, it will extol their virtues of being able to multitask well. The ugly truth is that the real definition of multitasking is starting many things without ever finishing anything.

Food for thought: Multitasking is much like the circus performer, spinning many plates at one time and rushing around to keep them all spinning.

Have you ever wondered the purpose of spinning all those plates ... it clearly takes lots of practice, but what is the real purpose of that? Busy being busy!

Today people like to emulate the image of the celebrity who has every minute of each day mapped out in advance. Somehow, we have all succumbed to this fast-paced, almost frenzied lifestyle. Every morning an "ALARM" goes off scaring you out of bed. You hurry around to get yourself and everyone else ready. You rush the kids out the door to either school or daycare. You fight the traffic on the way to work. You work through lunch to keep up with your boss' unrealistic demands. You attempt to leave on time to pick up your kids. You rush to soccer practice. You cram to get homework done. You struggle to get dinner ready. You set your "alarm," so you can dread having to do it all again in the morning. Your life is high pressure, high pressure, and more high pressure. You were never meant to be a pinball bouncing here and there and running around like a chicken with its head cut off. Being busy does not translate into a productive, healthy lifestyle.

What is the one day of the year that you get more done than any other day of the year? It is the day BEFORE you go on vacation. Right? That is usually the day that you get more done in 24 hours than any other time throughout the year. Why is that? Typically, it is because you HAVE to get everything that needs to be done finished in order for you to be able to leave.

Before vacation, you make a list of everything you must do, and you pointedly set out to accomplish everything on the list. You know what has to be done, you handle the distractions, and you are more productive than ever. How many of us spend more time planning our next vacation than we do planning our lives? To turn off the "Pinball Rally Stress Switch", you have to plan your day before it runs all over you.

If you manage your time, you will be amazed at how you can manage to get everything done. Once everything is done, a day of rest is in order for you. After all, even the Creator Himself only worked for six days and then rested on the seventh.

To turn off the "Busy Stress Switch" of being busy, here are our recommendations:

1. First, the next time someone asks you how you are, respond with, "I am blessed and not stressed." You will be amazed at how blessed and not stressed you will instantly feel. Simply saying those words out loud has a majestically freeing effect. The beauty of this is, the more you speak it, the more authentic it will become.

This is the first and easiest step to turning off the Busy Stress Switch.

2. Secondly, plan your day. Before going to bed, make a list of everything that really has to be done the next day. Once you make that list, prioritize it with the two things that absolutely "have" to get done, then list the things you would "like" to get done, and lastly, identify the two things that you can "eventually" get done. Begin your day getting those first two items off your list.

We recommend you write this list down so that you can physically mark them off as you go. That is a freeing process by itself.

Enjoy this step to becoming blessed and not stressed!

CHAPTER SEVEN
THREE MODES OF STRESS EFFECTS ON THE BODY

"Where is the panic button?!?" My boss yelled as he ran into the Art Department at work. "We have to have this project done immediately, if not sooner!" He was as high strung as a high-tension wire. Every project he brought in was always a chaotic situation. His behavior was a result of being mired in Chaos Mode.

There are three modes that people fall into based on their response to stress. They are Control, Chaos, and Collapse Modes.

CONTROL MODE

People who are in Control Mode tend to experience a low level of stress each day. They have turned off many of their Stress Switches and know how to utilize stress relief tactics to prevent any new stress from being stored in their body and negatively affecting their life.

When they do experience a stressful situation, as we all will at times, they immediately go into Control Mode and utilize a positive "Go-To," such as going to the gym, washing their car, organizing a closet, cleaning their home and or eating a healthy meal. By accomplishing a positive task, without anyone criticizing them, it is very gratifying and restores CONTROL to their life.

CHAOS MODE

People who are in a constant state of stress are in Chaos Mode. You can tell if someone is in Chaos Mode because they will have a Negative "Go-To." They usually can only manage their "Go-To" for a temporary "fix" of instant gratification that does not fix anything. They are only treating symptoms of stress, not the cause of the stress. They can't remember the last time they were even in Control Mode. They may spend money on things that they think will make their life less chaotic but seldom use these items. They rarely watch self-help videos (Reading self-help books would take too much effort) and get excited about bringing control back into their lives but lack the stamina to accomplish it. They can barely make it through each day, let alone take on a corrective program which, for them, would only add to their stress load, making things worse, not better.

When they experience (and they always do) a stressful day, they will automatically go right to their "Go-To," which is often some form of unhealthy or retail therapy. They will experience a very temporary rush of positive feelings only to feel worse when they wake up or get their monthly credit card bill. Rational thinking no longer exists, and this becomes their new normal. Their only escape is a temporary bandage that never results in less stress. Once they start to turn off their Stress Switches, they will be able to regain the composure and the energy to transition to Control Mode.

COLLAPSE MODE

People who have passed from Control and Chaos Modes are now mired in Collapse Mode. They have been in a stressed state for so long it has depleted their energy and hope. They have little motivation to do anything. It is all they can do to get out of bed in the morning. They are typically exhausted most of the time and need extended periods of rest even to feel like they can survive.

BRINGING BACK HOPE

If exposure to prolonged stress with no relief has caused the conditions mentioned above, only by turning off their Stress Switches, coupled with effective stress relief tactics, will they be restored to a state of calmness and control. If they allowed the stress to acclimate, they have the power to stop it.

A personal note from Matt:

One of my absolute heroes was my grandmother, "Mema." She was my hero for so many different reasons. However, her most amazing quality was that she was the most positive person I have ever known. If you had told her, "Wasn't it tragic how many people died with the sinking of the Titanic?" She was the type of person who would have said, "Oh yes, honey, it was just awful. But we should be grateful for all the people who lived." She exuded optimism! I talk about her in almost every speech or seminar that I give because of the way she chose to live her life. She passed away at the young age of 93, and I was blessed to help preach her funeral. Sadly, most people who live to be that old typically have a small funeral because they outlived all their friends. To complicate matters even more, my Mema retired as the manager of our local Department of Motor Vehicle. A 93-year-old who ran the DMV is someone we should have had to pay people to attend her funeral. However, at my Mema's funeral, it was standing room only!

As person after person walked by her casket to pay their respects, they told me what an incredible impact she had on their lives. They told stories about how she made them feel like they were the most important person in the world. They talked about standing in line longer so that they could have her help them. You could feel her love.

The sad reality is that she had every reason to be the most bitter, selfish person in the world. Her mother died at a young age, and she and her four siblings were raised by their father, who, in her words, "could be verbally mean." Not long after meeting my grandad, they "had" to get married, which was virtually unheard of in her day and time. Then, to put it mildly, my grandad was a very difficult man to live with. He could be everyone's best friend, but he could also be brutally tough to his family, especially when he drank. Don't get me wrong, I loved my grandad, but I don't respect the way he chose to live his life. Mema was the reason they had anything. She worked a full-time job and took care of everything at home. I say all that to say that my sweet little Mema CHOSE how she wanted to live. She had immense amounts of stress in her life but knew she was the only one who could control herself. She accepted and knew what she had to do to keep as many of her stress-switches turned off. In so doing, she left behind a legacy that many of us aspire to attain.

How can you handle the stress effects on your body?

STEP ONE

Understand you were created to live a blessed life, not a stressed life.

STEP TWO

Read and reread *Stress Free You*, and practice daily the principles in this book to help you rid your life of stress.

STEP THREE

Stress Free You will give you access to unique and useful stress relief tools, including the weekly Podcasts by Rich, Matt, and Matt's wife, Katy. Each week you will be able to benefit from a new podcast, focusing on Stress Switches and, more importantly, how to turn them off.

STEP FOUR

Enjoy your life FREE of Stress! Congratulations!

CHAPTER EIGHT

STRESS SWITCHES AND FIXES TO THE RESCUE

Imagine removing all the stress in your life with the flick of a switch. Wouldn't that be wonderful? What would your family, work, and social life be like if you could turn stress off that easily?

THERE IS HOPE!

You can actually remove all, and I do mean ALL, of the stress you deal with by turning off not just one but ALL of the "Stress Switches" in your life.

The number of stress switches you have to turn off depends on how many you have turned on.

Turning off Stress Switches is the backbone of *Stress Free You*. This brand-new approach is helping people from all walks of life, all over the world, and in countless situations live a stress-free life.

What makes these Stress Switches so amazing is that although the sources of Stress Switches vary significantly from the media, work, family, relationships, health, financial, they are simple and easy to turn off once you learn about them.

Because most of the stress you are facing is of your choosing, the good news is that you have the ability, the authority, and the choice to turn off your Stress Switches. That is why we wrote *Stress Free You*. *Stress Free You* will help empower you with the techniques for freeing your life of stress. This tool will show you how to turn off Stress

Switches and how to couple that with effective forms of stress relief.

Examples of Stress Switches and Fixes or How to Turn Them Off

Example 1: News Blackout

The news. Typically, is it the first thing we see in the mornings and the last thing we see at night. If it was just the news, or even fake news, that alone would be bad enough; however, 99% of what they report is terrible news. Human tragedies are an incredibly stressful way to start and end your day. In today's society, we are now inundated with the 24-hour news cycle. People have it blasting on their 200-inch TV's night and day. That is the equivalence of voluntarily immersing yourself in a septic tank and staying there. You absorb it, your kids absorb it, and it makes everyone negative, cynical, and critical. The reality is, what you focus on, you become. We are familiar with the harmful effects of second-hand smoke, but second-hand stress is just as dangerous.

Initially, the media just reported the news. They did not take sides, they did not choose sides, and they never criticized anyone.
In the 1960s, there were only 30-minutes of national news each night. Even then, those 30 minutes were viewed on a fuzzy 19-inch, black and white TV with rabbit ear antennas. By the time you add in commercials, it was only about 18 minutes of actual news. This was sufficient to cover any NEW news content that happened each day. Today we have 24 hours of people regurgitating that same 18 minutes of "new" news while yelling and screaming at each other.

The news outlets have gone a step further and have started taking sides in the political arena. This has further divided people. When you combine stressed out, passionate people with right or left-leaning talking heads, the result is a bunch of angry people (who should actually all be put in a timeout until they can get along).

The news almost always focuses on just the negative topics.

Rich said, "My neighbor Ed was in broadcasting, and he said, 'If a dog chases a man and bites him, that is not a story. But, if a man bites a dog, now that's a story.'" Negative, controversial stories of tragedy are the only course in the news diet.

The solution is simple. **"CLICK!"** Just stop consuming the news in any fashion. Turn off the news from every source, including TV, radio, printed, YouTube, news apps, websites, etc. Because, guess what is going to happen if something significant happens? Your friends are going to tell you.

Give yourself one week of a **News Blackout** and see how you feel. Flip the switch off. Stop consuming negativity. Enjoy a stress free, no news diet. Trust us; you're going to love it.

Example 2: 7th Haven

Before the Internet and mobile devices, when you left work, you could leave work. The only way for the boss to get a hold of you after hours was to call your one and only landline home phone from his one and only landline home phone.

When you were off, you were honestly off. This allowed you to relax, de-stress, and regroup for the next day. Including travel time, even if you worked around nine hours a day, you still had 15 hours of "off" time. That was a healthy ratio. Add in the weekend, and there was plenty of time to chillax.

Fast-forward to the excessively connected world of today and bosses are calling their employees at home, late into the evening, on top of sending emails and text messages almost 24 hours a day. The result of this is an increase in the stress load on the employee. This constant intrusion infringes into their family or relaxation time.

This keeps stressed-out employees in Fight, Flight, or Freeze versus Rest, Digest, and Restore mode.

It is essential to be a good employee and able to be contacted in case of an emergency. However, it is also essential to set up healthy boundaries. Some bosses respect an employee's time at home, but many other bosses may run a different schedule and will text or email employees at 2 AM. All this does is stress out the employee, so they have no rest time and end up going to work the next day already tired and stressed.

The Seventh Haven Stress Switch is the concept of not checking work emails or text messages from 7 PM to 7 AM, Monday through Friday. On the weekends, you can only check them sparingly if need be, but it is better if they are not checked at all.

Doing this will set the necessary boundaries that will allow you to turn off another Stress Switch. It will condition your boss and other coworkers that the only time to reach you is from 7:00 AM, during working hours, and up to 7:00 PM. This proactive maneuver will train them to contact you when it's appropriate, not because they procrastinated. Any other time, you're done for the day and in your Seventh Haven.

If you want to turn off the stress in your life, then start turning off the switches.

YOU deserve it. YOU were designed for it. YOU can have a stress-free life.

CHAPTER NINE

THE TOP 103 STRESS SWITCHES AND FIXES

We've included many of the most common stressful situations and suggestions to help you switch off your stress.

1. **News Black Out:** Stop consuming news in any fashion. The news is incredibly stressful.

2. **7th Haven:** Only view work-related messages between the hours of 7 AM to 7 PM.

3. **Be a Real Sport:** Stop watching sports and instead play them.

4. **Don't Show Me the Money:** Choosing a job with less stress, even if it has less pay, will pay significant dividends in the long run.

5. **Location. Location. Location:** Always keep your keys and wallet in the same place, so they are always easy to find.

6. **Don't Be a More-On:** Refrain from buying more and more stuff for instant gratification that will just leave you empty, with more stuff.

7. **Stop-Go Mode:** Turn off your Go, Go, Go work mode at home when you do simple things like chores and yard work. Enjoy the diversion from work and give your mind and everyone else a rest.

8. **Lick the Salt Habit:** Stay below the minimum daily amount of salt intake. This simple action will help keep your blood pressure low.

9. **H20 is the Way to Go:** Try drinking more water. Many people are walking around in a state of dehydration, which puts stress on their body's ability to function.

10. **Cool Vibes:** Only listen to relaxing music.

11. **Don't Touch that Dial:** Do not watch TV. Even if it is quality programming, the commercials will stress you out.

12. **Yell has the Fury:** Never yell at home or work. It is impolite and causes stress on those around you. Always treat your spouse like you treat your friends. The only time anyone should ever yell is if there is a real emergency.

13. **Go Green:** Slowly incorporate a large serving of green leafy vegetables into your daily diet helping you to enhance your immune system.

14. **The Cake is Fake:** Couples that are trying to both work and raise a family are trying to have their cake and eat it too. It may provide more money to buy "things," but it can also cause a much higher level of stress in the family. The two most important things a child needs are feeling love and having security. "Things" cannot provide that.

15. **The Parent Trap:** If you ask your child to do something, then the child should obey unless they can point out a significant reason why they should not. Do not cede control to your child and invite chaos into your home.

16. **The Best Place to Go-To:** When people are stressed, they turn to their Go-To. There are healthy and unhealthy Go-To's. Try swapping unhealthy Go-To's for more positive ones.

17. **Forgive and Forget:** Holding onto past pain is one of the most stressful things you can do. Choose to forgive, let go, and never mention it again.

18. **Fine Dining:** Eat more meals at home. They are much less expensive and can be better for your health.

19. **Don't Get Run Down:** Just because everyone at work is ready to run through a wall if asked, doesn't mean you should. Set your healthy boundaries.

20. **Healthy Vacations:** Go on vacations to relax, with little or no agendas.

21. **Touch it Once:** If you touch something, then either do it, file it, or toss it.

22. **Invest with Confidence:** Only check your investments once a year, on your birthday.

23. **Better to be an Hour Early than a Minute Late:** Strive to arrive early.

24. **Hooray for the Delay:** Treat delays as a blessing, not a stressing.

25. **Admit It:** When you make a mistake, and we all do, admit it right away. Covering it up adds a lot of stress.

26. **Chew on It:** Do as your mother told you and slow down when you chew your food. This action will give your system the ability to digest your food properly and prevent digestion issues.

27. **Commute Calmly:** Replace mindless radio with relaxing music or educational podcasts. Check out the *Stress Free You* podcast.

28. **Give Yourself Credit:** Only use a credit card if you can pay off the balance each month, protecting you from the high-interest rates they charge that are meant to enslave you financially.

29. **Have a Blast with a Fast:** Once a week, skip a meal. This will help you appreciate the meals you have and give you compassion for those who do not have enough to eat.

30. **Argue Not:** Never argue with anyone. When it comes to arguments, everyone involved is a loser, and it can cause collateral damage to others.

31. **Innocent Until Proven Guilty:** Do not use guilt to motivate people. It is very condescending and unproductive.

32. **Do a Random Act of Kindness:** Listen to your heart, and occasionally bless someone who is not expecting it. Pay for the person behind you at a drive-thru or a person struggling to pay for their groceries. Or possibly give a big tip to the people that serve you with thankless jobs like picking up your trash or delivering your mail.

33. **Hugs are Better Than Drugs:** Hug your family members at least once a day to show how much you love them.

34. **If You Complain, The Complain Will Remain:** Never complain.

All that does is magnify the problem instead of finding a solution to it.

35. **Swap Sweet for Savory:** There is a wide array of exciting and tasty savory flavors just waiting for you to try them. Many of them have actual health benefits where eating sugar has none.

36. **Peace Be with You:** Allow yourself to bask in at least 20 minutes of quiet time by yourself every day.

37. **Add Wait to Your Weight:** Do not weigh yourself more than once a month. People who weigh themselves every day are only adding to their stress.

38. **Be Right at Night:** Prepare for the next day the night before so to keep from being stressed first thing in the morning.

39. **Toxic Shock:** Try to eliminate any toxic friends who are negative or high maintenance.

40. **Safeguard Your Imagination:** Be careful what you watch. Your imagination is a large part of who you are and where your hopes and dreams are born.

41. **Sarcasm Leaves Scars:** Do not communicate with sarcasm. You are attempting to disguise how you feel in humor. It is not funny and is hurtful to the other person.

42. **Beat the Clock:** Try to refrain from looking at the clock constantly. Most of the time that keeps you stressed out and stuck in Fight, Flight, or Freeze mode. It affects your ability to be productive.

43. **Dare to Not Compare:** Never compare yourselves to others.

Instead, only compare yourself to YOUR OWN goals.

44. **Drop the Joystick:** Stop playing video games where there is always another level to attain and never win. Find a calmer board game or card game where you can have fun while playing.

45. **Watch what You Wear:** Wearing technology has many people continually checking every message that comes through, which never gives you a much-needed break from technology.

46. **Bolt the Jolt:** Caffeine does not give you energy. It stimulates your adrenal glands to produce stress hormones that can lead to adrenal burnout overtime.

47. **Take a Lunch Break:** People who are still in Go-Go-Go mode at work will be in Fight, Flight, or Freeze mode. That response was only designed to face danger, like running away from a lion. This mode shuts down your digestion system and sends its energy to your limbs and lungs. Not the right environment for digesting food. Don't eat at your desk. Go to the lunchroom or a quiet place to eat.

48. **That Sinking Feeling:** Always go to bed with a clean kitchen sink. Waking up to a pile of dirty dishes is a lousy way to start your day.

49. **Start a Wave:** As you walk around your neighborhood, take the time to wave at anyone as they pass by. It is a way to make someone else's day, and many of them will start waving back to you.

50. **Prime Time:** Only make important decisions when you are at your best. Not at the end of the day when you may be tired. Making the wrong decisions can have enormous negative ramifications.

51. **Pick Your Battles:** There may be times when you do have to fight for something you believe in, but try not to battle over the small stuff that typically does not matter.

52. **Dog-Gone:** Do not get a pet unless you can afford them. Pets need a lot of attention, only get one if you are committed to taking care of their needs every day.

53. **It Goes Beep in the Night:** Change the batteries on your smoke detectors every year. If not, it will emit an annoying tone, typically in the middle of the night.

54. **Circle Your Wagons:** Draw a circle around the three most important areas of your life. Eliminate everything that is not in your circles of importance. You can't do it all.

55. **Bet on Yourself:** Never gamble. It is very risky, and you have a slim chance of winning. Instead, invest the money in improving yourself.

56. **Wedding Bell Blues:** Do not spend a lot of money on weddings unless you or your daddy is loaded. Many couples blow a stack of money on a one-day event and struggle for the rest of their marriage financially.

57. **Photo Finish:** Every day before you go to bed, take a good look at the photos you have displayed in your home, making you more grateful for what's important.

58. **My Mother the Car:** Treat your car like you should treat your mother. Be kind to it, and make sure to provide what it needs to function correctly.

59. **Stop Spitting into the Wind:** Never bad mouth someone else or even talk negatively about them. It will always come back on you.

60. **Big Hello:** Greet everyone with a big hello. This makes them immediately feel welcome, and they will repay their gratitude.

61. **Penny-Wise and Pound Foolish:** Don't nickel and dime everything, which causes a lot of stress on everyone involved. After all, a penny saved is still only a penny. Be wise with your time.

62. **Rinse and Repeat:** Learn to enjoy even the tedious, repetitive tasks that we all have to do. Just put on some classical music and enjoy the time. Why get jacked up on stress when you are doing something that has to be done?

63. **Enjoy Thanks-Giving**: Start saying thank you to everyone you meet. You will be amazed at how well people will receive it. What you give out, you will get in return.

64. **Less is a Lot More:** Minimalism is a new trend that is freeing up a lot of people from extra costs and stressful decisions. They live in a simple home with only the necessary possessions—just another way to eliminate stress.

65. **Have a Moving Experience:** Once a year, pretend that you are moving and go through your entire home. Get rid of everything you don't need. Sell it, donate it, or toss it. Too much stuff will clutter up your life, causing unnecessary stress.

66. **Drop the Hammer:** Stop putting pressure on your family and people at work by threatening them with negative consequences. Negative motivation is negative.

67. **Be Unsociable:** Turn off social media updates that tend to interrupt your day. Only check your social media accounts for a few minutes per day.

68. **Waking Up Can Be Hard to Do:** Get out of bed slowly, and you will be able to stay in Rest, Digest, and Restore mode vs. jolting you into Fight, Flight, or Freeze mode. You are not a rabbit, so instead of hopping out of bed in the morning, try being the turtle and getting up slowly.

69. **Put Your Phone in Sleep Mode:** Find a place away from your bed for your cell phone so that it is not next to your bed while you are sleeping.

70. **Don't be Offensive about Your Defense:** Try never to defend yourself unless it is absolutely necessary. Defensive people are very negative and stressful to be around.

71. **Bitter Words Taste Bitter:** Only speak positive words that give life and not darkness. You never know who is listening, and all it does is empower the negative things in your life.

72. **People Pleaser:** It sounds nice to do things to please people, but the majority of people that practice this are only doing it because they want to be liked and not because they want to please the other person.

73. **Park Your Butt:** Go for a gentle stroll and find a place just to sit and ponder life.

74. **Arm Your Phone:** When it is safe, keep your phone at arm's length away, preventing you from looking at it always.

75. **Clean with Green:** Try using greener cleaners like vinegar in place of more cleaners with chemicals you can't pronounce. The cleaner the air in the home, the better for everyone.

76. **Two, Four, Six, Eight, it is Time to Delegate:** You are not superhuman. Delegate tasks at home and work to have everyone share in the load. "Many hands make light work."

77. **Shopping Pleasure:** Clean out your refrigerator and check your cabinets before going grocery shopping. This will save you money from buying items you don't need, and you will only get the things you do need.

78. **The Dinner Hour of Power:** Families that eat dinner together experience fewer issues with their children than those who don't. Enjoy the moments of time together.

79. **Feel like Crap, Take a Nap:** If you are tired, and if you are in a situation where you can, break for a few minutes to take a nap. You will be amazed how even a 15-minute nap can restore you to full power vs. struggling and making mistakes because you feel tired.

80. **It's a Question of Balance:** Refrain from checking your bank balance every day to see if you are overdrawn. Instead, find a way to manage your money better.

81. **Harden Your Soft Target:** Do not let stressed-out people dump their stress on you just because you are a family member or employee. Set up healthy boundaries.

82. **Take the Scenic Route:** Try going a different direction to work that may be more scenic, even if it takes you a few minutes longer. Just allow for the extra time and enjoy the drive.

83. **Clean Like Clockwork:** Schedule time each week to do your cleaning, laundry, etc. so you don't fall behind.

84. **Planning to Fail:** If you are not up to the amount of finances and time it takes to put on an event like a party or soirée, then refrain from doing it or make it much smaller. Only a few people have the skills necessary to pull off a stress-free event.

85. **Super Child Syndrome:** Many parents fall for the trap of having their kids involved in way too many activities. This stresses out their kids with the demanding schedule of parents driving them from one event to another. Let your kids be kids.

86. **Speak at Eye-Lovel:** Make eye contact when speaking with family members instead of looking at your phone or something else. Your family is supposed to be your object of affection, prove it.

87. **Say Nay to Tooth Decay:** What goes on in your mouth is a picture of the overall health of your body. Proper oral hygiene can save you tens of thousands of dollars later on in life.

88. **Take Care Before Sharing:** Only share relevant information with those who can handle it. Better to shield your children from things they have no control over and will only stress them out. Parents should NEVER speak about stressful situations in front of their children.

89. **Manage Up:** If your boss is unreasonable in their demands, then it is up to you to "Manage Up" and inform them of the

situation. If you do nothing, then you will get nowhere.

90. **Good Vibrations:** Sound is made up of vibrations. Even if we don't hear the noise, our ears pick up the vibration and convert it to sound. Many sounds can be stressful on the body. Try being gentler with everyday tasks like emptying your dishwasher, slamming the car door shut, banging a pot on the stove, etc.

91. **Timing is Everything:** Carefully consider the other person when you need to talk to them about issues. Try not to dump your cargo on a spouse the moment they walk in the door from a long hard day at work.

92. **Pay Yourself First:** Set up a regular automatic transfer from your checking account to a money market account that pays interest. This way, you pay the most important person first. YOU!

93. **Save for a Sunny Day:** Saving for a rainy day sounds depressing. Why would anyone want to do that? Save money in case you have an emergency; then, you will have the funds to cover it, making every day sunny.

94. **Auto-Matic Savings:** Cars cost a lot of money, and most people need them. Once you pay off your car loan, keep making the same payments to a separate bank account so you will have money for a down payment for your next car.

95. **Anger Management:** Try not to associate with angry people, if at all possible. They are stressed out people who are just venting. You could become like them if you are overexposed to them.

96. **Thrive with a Tribe:** One of the best ways to meet people with common interests is to join a group. It can be based on work, your hobby, or religious preference.

97. **Get High on Life:** Choose to de-stress by enjoying positive things like your loved ones and the wonders of the world we live in, versus things with lousy side effects.

98. **Know When to Say No:** Sometimes, you feel like you are being pulled into many directions at the same time with different commitments. Choose when to say no politely to any that will cause you to stress.

99. **Measure Twice, Cut Once:** Always check your work to make sure you did not overlook anything. Always strive to hand off an error-free project that you worked on.

100. **Tail Off:** Try not to tailgate the driver in front of you. It will stress them out and not leave you enough room to stop safely.

101. **Cause and Effect:** If you experience a health issue, look for the initial cause instead of just treating the symptoms.

102. **Shop Around:** Try only going through the outside aisles of the grocery store. That is where the majority of REAL food is located. The majority of the items in the middle aisles are usually highly processed foods that may not be the healthiest choices. This will save you money, time, and improve your health.

103. **Break the Mold:** Once in a while, mix your life up by doing something spontaneous. This will give you a fresh perspective on life and keep things interesting.

These are just the tip of the iceberg. Stay tuned for more Stress Switches to come by following us on social media, on our website at stressfreeyou.net, and on our Stress Free You podcast, available wherever you get your podcasts.

CHAPTER TEN
YOU CAN'T PUT A CORK IN A VOLCANO

From an outside perspective, a dormant volcano looks like a beautiful mountain stretching to the sky. Covered in lush green grass, towering trees, and flowering plants, it provides the landscape perfectly crafted for a destination vacation. It has an exterior that looks picture-perfect to the outside world. However, from somewhere deep within its lofty grandeur, something causes a change, and the internal temperature begins to rise. Initially, it's a gradual change. Eventually, one thing leads to another, and the temperatures start to increase at an alarming rate of intensity. Steam begins to build until the pressure causes cracks in the surface. The outside world notices the first signs of the growing internal problem as the steam begins to rise. Those closest to the source may not notice anything at all until the ground starts to shake as the picturesque landscape begins to fall apart. The internal temperature grows with an ever-increasing velocity to the point that the once vacation destination cannot stand the strain any longer. The volcano completely BLOWS ITS TOP! Boulders, steam, and ash explode into the sky! Lava bursts forth and rains destruction down upon anything and anyone in its path. No one is safe in any proximity of the tyrant. The volcano couldn't handle the internal pressure, lost its cool, and unleashed its fury.

Have you ever been the volcano? Have you ever been the victim of a volcano?

Life deals everyone a tremendous amount of pressure, struggles, trials, and problems. That is the nature of the world we live in. Consequentially, when you are exposed to stress over a prolonged period, it can build up an incredible amount of pressure both inside you and around you.

Without a way of releasing it, you will eventually have problems.

If you have ever experienced emotional trauma, it can create a devastating one-way door: a one-way door that lets the stress come in but seals it from going out. As the stress builds up pressure, without any natural relief, one day, the proverbial straw breaks the camel's back, an explosion of anger erupts, and the once-perfect exterior is changed forever.

Anger, like lava flowing down the mountain, follows the path of least resistance. That is why so many family members dump their anger on the ones they love the most. Those family members love us despite ourselves and will put up with it when others would never begin to tolerate the outburst.

On the surface, the angry person may seem to be suffering from some anger management issues. However, at the core, it is an inability to prevent and release stress that causes the destructive eruptions of anger.

Anger management classes might help but, addressing the emotional trauma and reducing the level of stress are the most effective treatments. Indeed, it is the only way to eliminate the build-ups that cause explosions.

THERE IS HOPE - *A hope that comes with a great deal of promise and peace.*

Approximately 90% of the stress you experience is of your own making. You have engaged countless Stress Switches, many of which are hidden in plain sight. The hope, promise, and peace come in knowing that YOU can control and make the changes to eliminate these Stress Switches.

Determine what turns your Stress Switches on and address those things immediately to keep the switches turned off. Doing so will keep the volcano cool, providing the beautiful, peaceful, and picturesque destination where you and your family deserve to live.

CHAPTER ELEVEN
HOW TO KEEP STRESS FROM MESSING WITH YOUR BRAIN

Your brain has been wired to operate in two ways: rationally and emotionally.

Consequently, your mind automatically adjusts based on each experience you face. For example, you are trying to assemble a piece of furniture that was delivered to you only a few hours before the company arrives.

It contains 123 parts that were manufactured in a foreign land, with instructions that were written in an impossible dialect. This has the potential to be a stressful situation. If you allow yourself to get stressed, then you force your brain to react emotionally to the stress, which causes your emotions to take over. That could cause you to shout things like, "I will never get this finished before they arrive!"

Without a doubt, when you let stress change how you are supposed to respond, you will experience an unbalanced life, causing countless problems. It can cause communication problems with your family. It can cause an internal battle in the brain that is almost impossible to win. It can cause productivity and communication problems at work. For example, every one of us has probably experienced the proverbial "Chicken Little" reaction when a co-worker comes running into the office saying, "The sky is falling! The sky is falling!" These overreactions can cause stress to spread to other co-workers, which affects the entire office environment.

Rich once worked with a woman named Mary. She was always

stressed out! She was persistently stuck in an emotionally stressed state of mind. Whenever the boss would do something that she did not agree with, she would storm into his office and say in her Southern accent that the boss was crazy and that she was going to quit. He would often remind her that she had already resigned before. Her response was, "Well, I will quit again!" After another reminder that she had quit twice, her response was, "Then I will quit again, and again and again!"

Her emotionally charged actions were a futile attempt to release stress. Had she stayed in the rational world, none of this would have happened. Stress can shrink, and often virtually erase your ability to think clearly, causing you to do things a sensible, rational person would never do.

Negatively speaking, whenever you live in a continued state of stress your brain can be rewired. Look at all the members of the military suffering from Post-Traumatic Stress Disorder (PTSD). While the majority of people in the military may not serve in a warzone, they can still suffer from continued exposure to stress that is piled upon them throughout their careers. To them, it becomes their new normal. This is why accepting the fact that mental issues are a real disorder is the first step to correctly rewiring the brain.

On the positive side, the "young lovers" will drive six hours each way to see the one who has stolen their heart and taken over their ability to think about anything logically. Or maybe it is the ones who will sit on freezing bleachers watching their athletic hero play a sport. Love is one emotion that can make people do crazy good things. For many in love, this becomes their new normal.

In the emotional state, your ability to focus and do even simple tasks is greatly diminished. Your emotions are there for a particular reason. They create your feelings. You laugh when you are happy, cry when sad, have compassion for those in need, and love others based on how well you relate to them.

To stay balanced, you need to keep the rational brain and the emotional brain in tune with each situation you face. The reality is that emotions and feelings will almost always dominate over facts and rational thinking.

To illustrate this, take Matt and his new wife, Katy. Katy was "venting" about something that had happened at work, which had really hurt her feelings. When she finished, Matt offered what he thought to be a rational response. She said, "I don't need the motivational speaker right now. I need you to listen." A rational response was not what she needed at the moment. She just needed to vent and get the issue out of her body. An emotional response will almost always win over fact. Emotional stress will overwhelm facts.

Has stress rewired your brain?

"The greatest enemy you will ever face is the one between your ears. YOU will do more to stop YOU than any other person on planet earth." –Matt Rush

Has stress caused your brain to short circuit to the point that the negatives overcome the positives? The best part of understanding and accepting this concept is the almost instantaneous freeing it brings your mind. Perhaps one of the easiest switches you can give yourself is by choosing to control your thinking instead of letting your thinking control you.

Reserve your emotions for the beautiful things that you were designed to give and receive. You are the boss of your brain!

CHAPTER TWELVE

HAS YOUR BRAIN BEEN HACKED BY STRESS?

From Rich:

When I worked in Bridgeport, Connecticut, I used to dread the brutally hot summer. On those days, whenever I would leave the cool, temperature-controlled climate of my office and walk outside, the oppressive heat and humidity would smack me in the face. The worst problem the heat caused me, was my constant need to pray that my car would start. It was a black, 1972 VW Super Beetle that did not like to start on sweltering hot days. Half the time, it would start with no problem, and the other half of the time, I would turn the key and get nothing but crickets. No sound at all.

The first time it happened, I got so mad that I pounded on the dashboard! Then I tried to start it again, and it started right up. So every time it would not start, I would beat the dash until it would start. Eventually, that stopped working, so I tapped around the steering wheel. Miraculously that worked, and I had a new trick to getting my car to start on hot days.

I finally took it to get checked out. The mechanic found the cause of the problem. It was a loose wire that would short out on hot days. Unbelievably, all it took was a short circuit, from one small wire, to shut down my entire car.

The toll that prolonged stress takes on the body and mind is devastating. People who endure long periods of stress are affected just like when a computer is hacked, in essence, by rewiring their brain. The once thoughtful, calm, rational person has been transformed into an easily agitated, highly irritable, and irrational person.

This prolonged exposure to being in "fight or flight or freeze" mode makes them feel like they are being threatened by almost anything. Even common-sense counsel from a trusted friend or family member can trigger an irrational response. This is because survival mode causes logic to become an evasive trait.

Stress is a powerful force that can vastly affect your behavior. When you are stressed-out to the point of being irrational, your critical thinking skills are significantly compromised. This can cause you to always be on the lookout for a shortcut, and unfortunately, the shortcut you end up with may cut yourself short by making poor decisions. If other people are aware that you are stressed and that your responses during those times can be controlled, then you are vulnerable to being manipulated. Which means someone can profit from your misfortunes.

You can tell when someone else is burdened with stress. Their "Go-To" goes south. For them, it is not the battle of the bulge, but the battle of the binge. They keep "bingeing" on unhealthy choices. This is where people are susceptible to being manipulated as they amp up their "Go-To" in order to meet the crisis. The illusion is to treat the symptoms, not fix the problems. Because their brains have been rewired/hacked by stress, they are at the mercy of the situation.

To fix the short circuits in your wiring, you must turn off the inflow of stress. Then, and only then, can the brain start the healing process.

CHAPTER THIRTEEN

WHY STRESS RELIEF IS NOT ENOUGH

A common definition of stress relief is, "Any act that aids in the relief of stress." Sounds easy enough, right? Besides, wouldn't you love to have some relief from your stress? Of course! Things like yoga, meditation, calm music, and exercise are all excellent examples of stress relievers.

The only problem is, you need a cure, not just relief! Like we said before, it would be like trying to drain your smartphone battery to zero while it is still plugged in. That would be impossible.

Stress relief by itself is not enough. Picture this:
If you are like most people, your stress level is probably at 85% and growing daily. Because of that you know you NEED some relief. Therefore, on your way home from a stressful day at work, you stop and indulge in an hour-long relaxation massage. This beautiful, peaceful hour seems to be precisely the stress relief you need. You feel every muscle in your body begin to ease. Your stress level has dropped to 75%. While that may not be a lot, you are just happy that it is moving in the right direction.

Your relaxed body melts into your car, and you begin the drive home. Then it happens. From out of nowhere, another stressed-out driver cuts you off and slams on their horn! To make matters worse, they display a hand gesture that proclaims that you are #1!

Boom! Now your stress level has blasted through the roof to 90% and growing!

If the world were as simple as puppy dogs and rainbows, then stress relief would be all you would need. Unfortunately, we all live in a fast-paced, stressed-out world. As long as you are plugged into the craziness, you will remain stressed.

According to mainstream medical experts, chronic stress is not something anyone in our society should take lightly.
Until you start to eliminate the source of stress, all the stress relief is just a temporary fix without making any long-term improvements. It is a flimsy bandage on a gaping wound.

That is why our revolutionary new concept of turning off Stress Switches is helping people.

Only when you begin to turn off each Stress Switch to stop the inflow of stress and then couple that with stress relief tactics to increase your outflow will you see any improvements. It is that simple.

That is why we have written this book. Imagine what your life would be like if every week, your stress levels were consistently dropping instead of rising?

Our bodies are like batteries that store stress. Unfortunately, whatever is stored will never be depleted unless you first stop the inflow. You could be 90 years old and still be saving the stress from when you were 12 years old, especially if you experienced a stress event that was coupled with emotional pain. Those events can be burned into your soul, such as parents announcing to their children that they were getting a divorce.

A personal note from Matt:

At the writing of this chapter, I am 46 years old. My parents divorced when I was in the 8th Grade. Even though that was many years ago, to this day, I can tell you about every detail of the night when my mom came in and told us kids that she and our dad were getting a divorce. I can still see what she was wearing, I remember what we kids were doing, and I can see some very precise details of that night. I can recall so much about that time period in my life that I dedicated an entire chapter to it in my personal book. This is why when emotional pain is combined with stress; it is exponentially more damaging.

You can go to all the psychologists and counselors you like, and they can help you identify the source of your pain. They can even help you talk about your pain. However, if the emotional pain is buried under layers of stress, it will rarely come to the surface, making it extremely difficult for anyone to help you permanently resolve and heal the pain. Additionally, if you are in a highly stressed state, you may not even have the mental or emotional capacity to deal with the buried pain.

What is so incredibly exciting about *Stress Free You* is that, as you turn off each of your Stress Switches, you will see your stress levels decrease. It will uncover the emotional baggage that has been buried for a long time and allow you to get the healing you finally deserve. When that happens, then you can drain stress out of your body with effective stress relief tactics.

From that point, you will be free of both physical stress and emotional pain, and can then truly accept that life is good.

CHAPTER FOURTEEN
PROCRASTINATORS CLUB

My mom said I wouldn't amount to anything because I procrastinate. I told her, "Just wait and see!"

Why do today what you can put off to tomorrow?

If good things come to those who wait, isn't procrastination a virtue?

I asked my friend what procrastination meant, and he said, "I'll tell you tomorrow."

The only good thing about being a member of the Procrastinators Club is that their meetings are always postponed until later.

Have you ever been guilty of putting things off that need to be done?

Of course, we all have. It's a trap that every one of us has fallen into from time to time. The real problem is when you put off those things that you NEED to do because you don't WANT to do them. This chapter was started with a few humorous one-liners to hopefully make you laugh. However, some incredibly stressful switches are turned on whenever you procrastinate.

The procrastinator always avoids difficult situations or tasks often while deliberately looking for distractions. It comes down to a lack of self-control that allows you to derail yourself instead of getting done what needs to get done. Your procrastination not only affects you but those you live and work with as well.

A note from Rich:

I was around 12 years old, and I remember pulling a neatly folded shirt out of my dresser. I tried it on and decided that I wanted to wear a different shirt. Now I was faced with a choice. I could fold the shirt and place it back in my dresser drawer, or I could throw it in my laundry basket. I choose the laundry basket. That meant that my mom had to carry my laundry with that perfectly clean shirt down two flights of stairs to the basement and put it in the washer, then the dryer and then back up two flights of stairs and fold it and place it back in my drawer. Sorry, Mom!

Could you be the "Perfectionist" who puts things off because it is a whole lot easier not to do something than to do it and have it fall short of your preconceived level of perfection? Therefore, your motto becomes, "It is better to not do it at all than to have it done less than perfect."

Or possibly, you let how you feel become the driving force of accomplishment. You may even use excuses like, "I just don't feel like doing it right now." However, then you don't "feel" like it tomorrow or the next week or the next month or the following year, and your feelings become an excuse for not doing what needs to be done.

Have you ever said, "I just work better under pressure"? Unfortunately, research has shown that this is not the case. Typically, that is just an excuse to put off what needs to be done.

In today's society, you are also surrounded by countless distractions, most of which are all at your fingertips. Your cell phone comes with a "Screen Time" feature. Your device will give you a report of how you spend your time staring at the screen. If you have an iPhone, you can swipe right from your Home screen to see your usage. Be prepared for what you are about to find. The results may shock you. The reality is that in the amount of time you spend on an electronic device, you could learn a foreign language, write a novel, organize your entire house and get more done than you have been accomplishing.

There are three types of procrastinators.

1. There is the "Thrill-Seeker" who likes to wait until the last minute in order to get the rush that it brings.

2. The second type is the "Avoider," who puts things off because of a fear of failure or even success.

3. Then there is the "Indecisive" procrastinator who can't make up their mind about anything.

At some point, you have probably been one of those three individually or possibly all at the same time. There is much stress created because of procrastination: internal stress, external stress, stress on relationships, sleepless nights, stomach ulcers, and the list can go on and on.

Procrastination at work

Does this sound familiar? The CEO of your company gives an assignment to the Vice President and with instructions that the assignment must be on the CEO's desk at 4 PM today. The VP rushes to the Head of the Department and offloads the task, saying that it is needed by 3 PM today. That Department Head passes the assignment off to the Manager with instructions that it is needed by 2 PM. The Manager hands it to the Coordinator and to be completed by 1 PM. The Manager assigns it to the employee who will do the job and with the directive that it is needed by noon. The only problem is that it is now 11:30 AM! The employee is super stressed trying to get the project finished in that short amount of time.

The point being, if you are in management, you need to plan so that your employees do not have to endure unnecessary stress. Your team should all understand this motto, "A lack of preparedness on your part does not constitute an emergency on my part." Be prepared. We have all heard the adage, "Those that fail to plan, plan to fail."

In the workplace, there is a certain "vacuum mentality" that thrives on the premise that once something is off your desk, you do not care about how it will affect others. The fact is, a business is only as strong as its weakest link in the chain. Successful companies create a culture that values every employee and does not burden them with unnecessary stress. Please understand that you are not expected to do everything correctly, but you are expected to do everything professionally. That's something that you can do instantly that will immediately begin to lower your stress. Remember, you handle animals, and you manage people.

Eat your frog in the morning!

The good news is that you can turn off the stress that is caused by procrastination. Mark Twain once said, "If the first thing you do each morning is to eat a live frog, you will have the satisfaction of knowing that it is probably the worst thing you'll do all day." How true is that? In other words, if you have something difficult to do in a day, do it first. Get it out of the way, so it isn't a mental drain on your soul.

Some people are also guilty of continually saying, "There is never enough time to get everything done that I need to do!" Guess what? If that is your attitude, there probably never will be. Successful people don't try to do everything. They learn to focus on the most critical tasks and make sure those get done. They do the hardest or most important before any other.

Here are a few suggestions to help you overcome procrastination:

1. Set specific and achievable goals for yourself.
2. Break those goals down into incremental steps.
3. Plan your day in advance.
4. Apply the 80/20 Rule, which says that 20% of your effort will give you 80% of your results.
5. Identify your time wasters.
6. Have others hold you accountable.
7. Create effective rituals for using your time.
8. Set specific times/dates to have something accomplished.
9. Prioritize the first, second, and third most important things for you to accomplish in a day.
10. Be prepared before you start anything.
11. Anticipate obstacles.
12. Motivate yourself.
13. Declutter your life.
14. Finish what you start.
15. Reward yourself for accomplishing a task.

To create a stress-free life, you have to cancel your membership in the Procrastinators Club.
Enjoy the feeling of not waiting until the last minute.
Deny fear and choose success.
Be confident in your God-given abilities.

The immediate sense of accomplishment will be a gratifying sensation that will lead to a Stress-Free You!

CHAPTER FIFTEEN
THE MAD RUSH

A personal thought from Rich:

Regardless of what you think about this chapter title, I am not calling my Co-Author, Matt Rush, insane. However, he can be insanely funny.

Instead, I am referring to the insane pace many people live their lives: the mad rush.

When people are checking their work emails while they go to the bathroom, you know that life is moving way too fast! Is there nowhere left for a moment of stress-free peace?

For most families, the stress starts early every weekday morning:

- You're yelling at your kids, "Hurry up, or you will be late!" STRESS!
- You rush them out the door and race to get them to school and you to work on time! STRESS!
- All-day on the job it is non-stop! STRESS!
- You leave as soon as you can to rush to pick up the kids and race home to throw a dinner together. STRESS!
- Then it is yelling at the kids to hurry up and finish their homework so that they can go to bed. STRESS!
- You virtually pass out at night, exhausted from the stress of the day, and the stress of knowing that you get to do the same mad rush all over again tomorrow. MORE STRESS!

During the week, there never seems to be quality time anymore. You typically live all week with the only hope of having some downtime on Saturday. However, Saturday finally gets here, and it is booked solid with rushing the kids to activities like soccer and dance and playing catch up from everything that you didn't get done during the week. STRESS!

That gets you to "Segregated Sunday," with the women doing one thing and the men yelling at the game on TV. While in the back of your mind, you're thinking about how much you dread the crazy week to come. STRESS!

Fast forward twenty years and two tired, worn-out parents will remark, "Where did all the time go? It was just a blur."

It is almost impossible to have a good, quality family life during the child-raising years if it is continuously spent doing the mad rush.

Kids get it

Kids understand how slow time passes. For example, "Are we there yet?" "How much farther is it?"

A note from Rich

Years ago, my super wife was working nights at the hospital as an RN. As she came home in the morning, I left to go to work at my day job. Our two kids were at the age that they could be OK not being watched during the day while mom slept. The first morning that Donna came home from working nights, I told Sarah and Stephen, "Here is the number to my office. Call me if you need anything." However, then I sternly told them, "DO NOT, I REPEAT, DO NOT EVER, NO BUT NEVER, WAKE YOUR MOM UP!"

I arrived at work at 8 AM and dove headfirst into my workload, thinking that the kids will do just fine. In a few minutes, I received a call from our receptionist, who sheepishly said that I had a call from Stephen Taylor.

I told her I would take the call and answered it, "Hi Steve, are you OK?"

He answered, "Dad, it's 8:21." I replied, "Thanks Steve, keep quiet and do not wake mommy. I will talk to you later. Bye." I went back to work only to have the receptionist buzz me again, saying there was a Stephen Taylor on the phone for me. I took the call, and Stephen said, "Dad, it is 8:23." I replied, "Thanks for letting me know and do not wake mommy up. Bye."

Guess what happened next? You got it! Two minutes later, four minutes later, seven minutes later, he called back again and again just to let me know what time it was.

Time was moving very slowly for my son. Honestly, that is how we are supposed to experience the passage of time, not in a mad rush every day.

The good news is that you are now in the right place because *Stress Free You* will help you discover your resolution to the mad rush.

It has been said countless times that one of the biggest obstacles facing the family right now is over-commitment; time pressure. There is nothing that will destroy family life more quickly than hectic schedules and busy lives, where spouses are too exhausted to communicate, too worn out to have sex, too fatigued to talk to the kids. That frantic lifestyle has the potential to be highly destructive.

For some reason, society has sold you that, "Busy is the new happy."

Yet, is it?

For most of you, I would dare to say that being in the mad rush feels a lot more like you are slowly drowning in the pile of busy. For most, it has become overwhelming. Kids today have been conditioned to a fast-paced lifestyle to the point that there can be no downtime.

A note from Matt

First, I'm so glad that Rich doesn't think I'm insane, and I do have a few jokes that I would love to share.

Secondly, Rich's story goes right to the point that we want to make. Being in a constant rush is not how we are supposed to use our time. For example, have you ever studied a clock? Seconds tick off one by one. You were even taught to count every second slowly, one Mississippi, two Mississippi, three Mississippi, and on and on. **Time is supposed to be measuredly invested, not frantically spent.** How do you usually spend yours?

I understand what some of you are probably saying right now, "Yeah, but they don't understand my life and my schedule." You are correct; we do not know your schedule. However, we do know that nine out of 10 people are overly involved and over-committed.

My sweet wife Katy and I are not blessed with children, but because of my older brother and younger sister, I am Uncle MattMatt, and she is Aunt Katy to a niece and three nephews, Rachel, Staten, Jarett, and Brik.

As I have watched the kids grow up, I have marveled at how "busy" they are! Not only during the school year but also during the sacred summer months that are now packed with non-stop activities. At the end of one particularly busy summer, my sister said that her two boys had only had two weeks where there was nothing to do. Their most requested activity had become, "Can we just have a stay home day?"

Last summer, she said her mission was to let them get bored. There were only two scheduled items on the agenda for the summer: swimming lessons and church camp. Television was limited to mornings only. All electronic devices had timers on them that would shut them off at the predetermined time. The only way the boys could get more than the allotted time was by doing certain "chores." She found the list online, but some of the chores involved reading for 45 minutes, exercising, going swimming, making their bed, folding their laundry, or being outside for one hour, etc. It was a little difficult at first, but ultimately it was fantastic! Once the expectations were set, explanations made, the boys knew what they could and couldn't do every day. They even started holding each other accountable. When one of them would say, "I'm bored." The other would say, "Go do something on the list." It is about managing the clock vs. letting the clock control you.

To further prove the point that we are all in a mad rush, how many of you have said, "I just don't have enough time"? Oddly enough, every day has the same amount for every one of us. Each day has 86,400 seconds, no more, no less. One of the exercises that are often done in our live training events is to have the attendees name the five most essential things in their lives. I always say that "If you have five kids don't list them all! Just give me the five categories of the most important things in your life." Can you name your top five?

The great news is that we all know each other better than you think we do because I can name most of what you put on your list. I call them the **Five F's**: Faith, Family, Friends, Finances (your career), and Fitness (health). How did I do with yours?

Typically I can get most of them.

However, without fail, I know one thing that is on every person's list, and that is "Family." Virtually every person on planet earth will list family as one of the essential things in their lives. So then I ask the question, "How much time did you spend with your family in the last week?" Clarification, "How much *unobstructed* time did you spend with your family?"

The reality is that I can typically calculate that in minutes. You probably instantly disagreed with that calculation. However, if I said that TV time doesn't count, sporting events don't count, sitting in the same room, but staring at different devices doesn't count, making a mad dash from one activity to the next doesn't count, etc. The only thing that counts is how much one-on-one, unobstructed, personal time did you spend with your family? How many family meals did you have together? How much time was spent just talking to your spouse or your kids? Isn't it a scary thought?

Thirty years ago, it was eight hours per week. Twenty years ago, it was six hours per week. Ten years ago, it was three hours per week (or 25 minutes per day). Today the average parent now only spends seven minutes per day in communication with their kids. That is a SHOCKING number! I understand that everyone is "busy", that is life. However, has society conditioned you to be busy for the sake of being busy? There are 1,440 minutes in a day. Even if you take away sleeping and work and school, there are still plenty of opportune minutes lost every day to being in the mad rush.

The point is, you just said that one of the essential things in your life is your family and yet you can calculate the time spent with them in only minutes per week. To those closest to you, love is spelled, T-I-M-E.

There is hope!

A few suggestions to get out of the Mad Rush with the ones we love:

- How different would your day be if you started each morning by gently waking up instead of going off to an "alarm." **Rest.**
- Be an active listener more than a constant speaker. **Listen.**
- Use open-ended questions like, "What do you think..." "Why do you think..." "What would happen if..." **Probe.**
- Commit specific time to spend with the ones who mean the most to us. **Invest time.**

The question is, "Why?"

A personal note from Matt:

When I was the CEO of a large organization, I lived five hours away from the place I call "home." During those days, I would come home on weekends as often as I could. However, my time was largely consumed by the day-to-day operations of the organization. Also, as often as possible, I was traveling around the country speaking and training.

On one rare weekend, when I was home visiting family, my then seven-year-old nephew Jarett asked, "Uncle MattMatt, did someone make you take that job you have?"

I responded confidently and probably somewhat indignantly, "Well, NO."

He looked me in the eyes and said in the most serious and inquisitive voice, "Then why would you take a job that takes you away from your family so much?"

You could have knocked me over with a feather. Out of the mouths of babes come great truths. I had let the urgent replace the important. It was at that precise moment that I quit my job. Internally initially, but I began to take steps to vacate my corner office, leave my role as CEO, and get back to what was important.

I know I could still do even better; we all can. However, as I am writing my part of this chapter, I am so thrilled to tell you that last night, two young boys, ages 14 and 10, who call my wife and me, "Aunt Katy and Uncle MattMatt" rode their bikes to our front door, just because they wanted to say hi. That is living the life of the important.

Every day slowly ticks away, leading seconds to minutes, minutes to hours, hours to days, days to months, months to years, and years to eternity. The story about how you live your "dash" is a poignant reminder of what is truly important. On your tombstone, there will only be two dates, your beginning, and your end. The only thing that matters is how you live the dash in between those two dates.

So I ask this question, are you frantically spending or measuredly investing your time?

Invest your time wisely. The seconds may tick by slowly, but life is racing by. There is a scripture that says, "Life is but a vapor that only appears for a little while and then vanishes away."

Get out of the mad rush and soak in the presence of a stress-free day.

"Time will take the days off the calendar; only you can fill the days." –Matt Rush

CHAPTER SIXTEEN

FLEE THE "STRESS FLEAS"

Stress is like the wind; you may not be able to see it, but you can certainly feel its effects pressing against you.

Stress is like a bolt of lightning. It flashes out of nowhere and damages whatever it strikes.

Stress is like a flea. It takes up residence in your body, draws from your soul, multiplies, and continuously looks for another person to inhabit.

When you experience negative emotions, it is usually caused by a stress flea burrowing into your body.

Individuals who are completely infested with "stress fleas" can walk into a room full of happy, cheerful people and instantly start to change the dynamics of the room. They begin by trying to engage other people in a "discussion" with the infectious intention of escalating the conversation into an argument. Being right or wrong is not even an essential factor in the argument; they just need to unload their stress.

These individuals may not consciously be aware of their actions, but their minds are desperately trying to unload as many "stress fleas" as possible to gain the slightest amount of relief. They seem to have the uncanny ability to tap into some dark places and come up with the perfect words to start an argument. After all, misery almost always loves company.

Countless people have been unknowingly drawn into an argument by people loaded with “stress fleas.”

Even worse than the “flea infester” is the person who can transfer stress as fast as lightning!

From Rich:

I cautiously extended my finger toward the finger of the other Cub Scout. Before our fingers even touched, there was an audible crack from a colossal spark! Amazingly, our fingers never touched, but the charge of static electricity arced from his finger to mine. WOW, did it hurt!

Forty Cub Scouts, including me, were running around the altar area at St. Rose of Lima Catholic Church in Short Hills, New Jersey. One of the scouts realized that scuffing their leather shoes on the thick red carpet produced static electricity, and we all started scuffing and zapping each other!

This random activity is what bored 8-year-old boys do when left unsupervised. The President of the United States could have been that night’s special guest, but all I can remember is how empowering it was to scuff our feet, sneak up behind someone, zap them on the back of their ear, and hear them holler from the shock!

We were unloading a harmless stored charge of static electricity. This shocking method is the same way people unload their stored stress on each other. Yes, people store and release stress in the same manner.

When people with stored stress come in contact with each other, it can work much like trying to put a plug into an outlet. A spark jumps from the outlet to the plug before it’s even plugged in. That is called “arcing” and occurs whenever electricity is discharged along an unintended path. They may even be thought of as negative or filled an anger problem, but in reality, they are overwhelmed with stress and are desperately trying to drain it from their bodies.

Often, when someone is maxed out from a stressful day at work, they will "arc" with the first person that is unsuspecting enough to engage them. Like a moth drawn to a flame, the stressed person will start a rational discussion to lure the innocent victim into an argument. The argument almost always, escalates drastically and causes the stress to "discharge" along an unintended path.

In addition, whenever you are dealing with a negatively charged, stress-flea infested person, do not even hint at anything that might be negative or critical. The stressed person will take an inch and turn it into a mile. Remember, they don't care about the discussion; they just want to unload. They will occasionally even use provocative words to lure you into a debate. One minute, you are peaceful and in a good mood, and before you know it, you're in a full-blown, rip-roaring argument! Later you might even find yourself scratching your head, saying, "How did this happen? What a shock that was!"

Even though, your natural response is to defend your beliefs and yourselves, do not fall for this trap. Never, never, never argue with anyone. No good will come from it. The expression "winning an argument" is a sham. It takes two to argue, and it always produces two losers. Arguments are virtually always stress-induced. They are emotionally charged moments that someone is attempting to disguise as a rational form of conversation.

A note from Matt:

One of my favorite professors in college was a man by the name of David Vernon. We called him "Brother Dave." After college, I spent three years working at the university. During that time, Brother Dave and I became very close friends. I adored his entire family.

On April 15th, 2005, at the age of 51, Dave passed away from a brain aneurysm. Obviously, we were all shocked and devastated.

Hubert and Faye were his parents, and I had come to love them like my own grandparents. For years after Dave's passing, I would call them on Christmas Day just to check in on them to wish them a Merry Christmas. In addition, anytime I was passing through their hometown, I loved stopping in for a visit. Now that they have both passed on as well, I truly treasure those moments that we spent together.

Hubert had passed away a number of years before I met and married my wife, Katy. However, after we got married, we were often able to stop and visit with Faye. Because Hubert and Faye were childhood sweethearts who had spent close to 70 years together, as newlywed's, I wanted her advice. I asked what her what their secret to a successful marriage had been. Faye said without hesitation, "We never argued. Whenever I wanted to get upset and worked up about something, I would really start telling him about it. After I would finish my spat, Hubert would always put both his hands on my shoulders, look at me with a sweet smile and say, 'And I love you too, dear.'" She said, "You know, it really is hard to argue by yourself. That was why we loved each other so much for so long."

When dealing with people who have become infested with stress or allowed it to build up in their bodies, you only have two options:

Option one: do what you can to avoid them and not engage with them.

Option two: give them unconditional love. This kind of love is the antithesis to "stress fleas" and the negative electricity that these people carry. Approaching them with love is the only way to calm a storm and shield yourself.

Indeed, it is impossible to argue by yourself. I believe that Faye's advice is the best advice that any of us could take to heart. If we all lived like that, stress would flee from us and our lives would be filled with love.

CHAPTER SEVENTEEN
WHATEVER YOU FOCUS ON YOU SERVE

"Is that flame real? Let me touch it. Ouch! That hurts!" This reaction is what happens when you combine curiosity with ignorance.

From Rich:

That was me when I was five years old. Full of curiosity! This event took place in 1960, where the simplest of things would amaze us, kids, for days. Back when our attention had a span!

My older brother Wally had just gotten a magnifying glass and had focused the rays of the sun onto everything in sight. A leaf, an unfortunate bug, twigs, etc. It made a tiny little flame that amazed us all. Even though my brother's magnifying glass was no larger than 4 inches in diameter, it harnessed the power of the sun millions of miles away.

That is the extreme power of focus. The same way the magnifying glass captivated our freckle-faced gang of kids, what we give our attention to becomes our world. It can consume us if we give it our power. It becomes our focus.

Now think about the last time you had pain of some kind: a headache, a throbbing tooth, a sore back, or even a rash from Poison Ivy. You will appreciate my next experience!

While living in Connecticut, Hurricane Gloria knocked down a large red oak in my neighbor's yard. Since I had a fireplace, I asked them if I could have the wood. They agreed, and I had a guy cut the tree in sections.

When the wood was all cut, I bare-armed hauled one large section of the tree after another into my yard to be stacked and split. Unfortunately, I did not notice that Poison Ivy vines were growing along the trunk. As we had already had a frost and the leaves had dropped, there were "no three leaves and shiny" for me to see.

I'll bet you know what's coming next!

Sure enough, the next day, I awoke with both my forearms wholly covered in a horrifically, itchy rash. To make matters worse, it was a Sunday, and the doctor's office was not open.

I tried everything I could, but I could not stop scratching. It consumed my every thought!

On Monday, I went with my pregnant wife to her appointment with her Gynecologist. While there, I asked her Gynecologist if he would write me a prescription for my rash. He agreed, and the combination of the steroids and ointment worked wonders. (That was in the 1980s, so I am not sure if an insurance company of today would agree to pay for a man getting a prescription for Poison Ivy from a Gynecologist.)

Needless to say, while dealing with that rash, my mind was fixated on only one thing, RELIEF. Our bodies are automatically designed to find relief from our mental and physical problems.

If you are always under stress, you will be forced to serve that stress. You will be compelled to find relief from the stress. People may boast that they can handle stress, but in reality, that is like holding flaming balls of fire in your hands. At best, all you will be able to do is juggle them, causing you even more stress.

Stress will narrow your focus to the point that all you will be able to see are your problems. Even though solutions may be nearby, if they are not within the frame of your magnifying glass, you will never see them.

Many people are being consumed by stress every day. They say things like, “No rest for the weary!” Their lives are in a downward spiral, with their only hope being that someday things will get better. The problem with this approach is that over time things don’t get better; they just get bitter from all the pressure.

Stressed out, people learn to embrace stress as their lifestyle. This approach is dangerous. Acceptance is not relief. It’s like bringing a momma Grizzly bear into your home while you are messing with her cubs. Stress can and will overpower and consume you.

Just remember, stress relief by itself is not sufficient. It is like charging into a burning building carrying a water pistol!

To achieve freedom from this “stress mess,” you need to change your focus by switching off the sources of your stress. That will allow you to shift your “magnifying glass” to things that will benefit you. Then you can genuinely enjoy love, joy, peace, a sound mind, and a stress-free life.

Let *Stress Free You* replace your water pistol!

CHAPTER EIGHTEEN
I FEEL GOOD!

Your happiness baseline should be on the plus side of joy every day.

We are designed to have and enjoy love, joy, peace, kindness, patience, and self-control. Do you know that relaxing feeling of taking a hot shower or soaking in a bath? That is how you are supposed to feel as you go throughout your day. Any straying from that core of goodness is a sign you need to adjust.

Going through life can provide temporary physical challenges, like catching a cold, injuring an arm, or enduring emotional challenges. These are mostly short-term challenges, and the body has built-in repair mechanisms to heal itself of the problem.

For most people, high-stress levels will rob them of any chance of finding joy. Therefore, if you are not feeling joy in your life, you need to evaluate what is causing the problem.

Just because you live in a world of stress does not mean you have to succumb to it. You are only supposed to feel stress for a matter of minutes throughout your entire life. Those times of stress are reserved for rare occasions when fight or flight are necessary for survival. We are not supposed to experience stress for prolonged periods.

The process of stopping the inflow of your stress will allow stress relief tactics to increase the outflow of stress from your body. Together these two steps will help you maintain a stress-free life.

It will feel so good to sit back and enjoy your “stress” fading away.

CHAPTER NINETEEN
DEADLINE PRESSURE COOKER AND BEYOND...

From Rich:

From the 1950s and into the early 1970s, there were virtually no deadlines in business. There were time frames of when you had to finish projects, but your boss gave ample time to do the work.

However, the only exception was the advertising business, which is my chosen profession. When I was assigned a project, I would always ask the proverbial question, "When do you need it completed?" The commonly known answer was still, "Yesterday!"

That "last minute" mentality stayed out of the rest of the business world UNTIL 1971 when Federal Express (FedEx) started their overnight delivery service. Before Federal Express, the only way to send anything was through the US Postal Service, which took at least a couple of days, if not more. On the rare occasion that you were desperate, you could buy an expensive plane ticket, fly it to your destination yourself, and then fly back home.

I remember very clearly all the managers of the company where I was working talking about the benefits of Federal Express. They could now procrastinate until the last minute and still make deadlines. This approach just made them less efficient managers. It made everyone else in the chain less efficient because of the added pressure. There were times when the managers would come into my art department and say, "I need 'X' done by the end of the day so we can 'FedEx' it to the printer by tomorrow." I suppose that it was likely that they had a rush of power knowing that they could pull off this last-minute project. The "rush" they were experiencing was a temporary high from the stress. The problem is that stress in any form is harmful.

Sidebar observation: Over the years of being a graphic designer, I have done thousands of projects, and many have been last minute. I have always found it somewhat amusing that others may have had two weeks to work on it, but the graphic designer and the printer still got two days to make it happen.

Indeed, there are good things about the overnight shipping business, but like anything, it can make some bosses lazy, thus forcing their stress on their staff.

The moral of the story

If you have a "Last-Minute Manager" who gets a rush out of pushing things to the limit, then you will need to learn how not to get caught up in their stress. Otherwise, it will put you into a "flight or fight or freeze" mode, which will vastly reduce your creativity and problem-solving abilities. After all, no one can work to the best of their ability when they are under that kind of pressure.

Warning, Nerd Fact: The cerebral cortex is the part of our brains where reasoning, thinking, planning, and rational decision making happens. When we are under stress, the part of our brain called the Amygdala automatically activates the fight or flight or freeze response. This action transforms the highly qualified employee into someone fighting for survival and greatly diminishes their ability to function at their optimum level.

And if you are a Manager, do not squeeze your staff with last-minute pressure. When you can minimize their stress, they will not only become a real treasure to you, but you will also become a real treasure to them, and then you can both live stress-free lives.

And beyond

Beyond the pressure cooker, some managers will use implied stress to try to motivate their employees. They will hint at the importance of a project and the consequences if it does not go well.

When they say, “It better go well or else.” What they mean is:
“If this flops, then we will have cutbacks.
No more free coffee, salary freezes, outsourcing to India, and
you won’t be able to pay your phone bill!
You will turn out to be rude, crude, inhumane,
and you won’t even be able to afford to take your kids to Burger Doodle.” That is using implied stress — saying words with an inflection in their voice, emphasizing the “heaviness” of the situation. This approach adds a tremendous amount of stress on the employee, shifting them into “fight or flight or freeze” mode, which in turn shuts down their creative and critical thinking abilities.
The managers’ thinking is that this is important and important needs SUPER motivation. They are using a stick to “threaten” employees, putting them into survival mode. When people are in danger, they cannot think clearly.

Managers and supervisors who use implied stress as motivation are not effective bosses. Their actions shift unnecessary strain on the employees, creating an atmosphere that no one enjoys. Using positive reinforcement as much as possible is very important. Psychologists say that it takes nine positives to overcome one negative.

Parents can unknowingly do the same thing when they condescendingly say something like, “Did you do your homework tonight?” What they mean is, “If you don’t do your homework, then you won’t get good grades.

Without good grades, you're not going to get a scholarship to college. If you don't get a scholarship to college, you will have to live with your parents for the rest of your life.
You'll end up getting a dead-end job, marrying a loser,
having wacko kids, driving a beater of a car that breaks down all the time, never having any fun, and living a miserable, wretched life.
All because you didn't do your homework." Whew!

Obviously, that is an exaggeration, but every stressed person has a "Dump-On." When their pressure builds to a point where it can no longer be contained, they will eventually release it on their "Dump-On." These are often soft targets like coworkers, spouses, children, or even the family dog.

Stress can manifest itself in various ways, such as physical or emotional abuse. Many extremely stressed people have been prescribed prescription drugs and spend hours in therapy and counseling. Often they focus on the symptoms instead of lowering their stress levels, which is most likely the culprit.

In the workplace, stress often causes bosses to be overly critical; resulting in them overworking their employees, or yelling and embarrassing them, which causes these employees to suffer from **the boss's** stress relief.

These stressed-out bosses are just bullies with a different name. Just as with all bullies, the only effective way to manage them is to set up boundaries. You must tell the offending person that you understand they are stressed out, but they are not to dump on you.

If you are the offender, you should be aware that there are measures to help you switch off your stress. A temporary measure would be physical activities such as working out, playing a sport, dancing, etc..

These activities will help to redirect your stress away from others.

An extreme example is two boxers who stand toe to toe for 12 rounds, trying to knock each other out, only to end up hugging each other at the end of the fight. That is a benefit of physical exertion to expend stored stress. You release it from your body. From a physical standpoint, your body also expels stress hormones when you sweat. So, sweat it out.

The only way for a person to not have a Dump-On is not to be stressed out in the first place. This level of tranquil life is achievable as you start to lower your stress levels on your way to experiencing your stress-free life.

Stop adding unnecessary pressure and creating challenges for achievement.

Stop thinking that implied stress is a motivator and use realistic goals with specific outcomes. Stop adding stress to an already stressful world.

You deserve a stress-free life; other people are crying out for it; students need it. Life is tough enough; don't be the cause of making it tougher.

Start becoming part of your solution. Start taking steps to turn off your stress switches and begin living a stress-free life. People will see the change in you, and they will want it too! From corporate executives to small business owners, from teachers to stay at home moms, manual laborers to tech gurus, retired individuals to current students, we ALL deserve a stress-free life. Quite frankly, we all need it! Life is tough enough; don't be the cause of making it tougher.

CHAPTER TWENTY
FATHER PANIK VILLAGE

From Rich:

There was a housing project in Bridgeport, Connecticut, called Father Panik Village. It was built in 1939 and, over the years, slowly degraded into a slum. It became a place where drugs and crime were rampant. At one point in my career, I worked in Bridgeport but lived in the neighboring town of Fairfield. There was a saying that we all knew, "NEVER go into Father Panik Village." If you did, you might not come out alive. It was a rough place.

Most people who panic when faced with stress is because that is what they have done in the past. This becomes a "normal" way of responding to stress.

Typically, when someone panics, the first thing we usually say to them is, "Don't panic." Yet when has that ever worked? When a person panics, he/she is entirely thrown into the "Fight or Flight or Freeze" mode. At that point, almost all of their reasoning flies out the window, making people susceptible to being manipulated or exploited. Desperate people will do desperate things. They immediately turn to their "Go-Tos." They may do a lot of things that are not in their best overall interest, such as impulse spending, consuming unhealthy foods, and even risky behavior.

At this point, we must ask, "What are your "Go-Tos" in these situations? Keeping a clear head only comes from not being overloaded with stress. When a situation arises, you know how to react to ensure you make the right decisions calmly.

An anecdote from Rich:

My brother Tom told me a remarkable true story. He had a classmate of his at the University of Rhode Island who was pledging to join his fraternity. He was blindfolded, driven around for hours, and then left on a road at night that was lined on both sides with dense woods. It was his responsibility to make it back to campus without any money or transportation.

His friend was thrust into the perfect opportunity to panic. Instead, he calmly surveyed his surroundings. After his eyes adjusted to the night, through the woods, he noticed something peculiar and started walking towards it. He walked past his old tree fort and directly into the backyard of his parent's home. His parents were a bit shocked but gladly welcomed him into the comfort of home. He sat down to an excellent dinner and laughed about his good fortune. He slept in his bed that night, and after a hearty breakfast, they drove him back to school.

Moral of the story, my brother's classmate would have missed all this if he had panicked!

In 1994, what had once been a dream housing project for many had become a criminal paradise, and sadly, Father Panik Village was vacated and demolished. Father Panik Village became known as a place where dreams became dust.

Don't let stress cause your dreams to turn to dust.
Develop healthy "Go-Tos." Stay out of Father Panik Village.

Staying stress-free is the only way to be.

CHAPTER TWENTY-ONE

NEEDING A VACATION FROM YOUR VACATION

COWABUNGA! You are finally on vacation!

It has been a super stressful year, and it is time for a major va-ca-tion! Since you only get one week off a year, you jam-packed the entire seven days full of exciting fun-filled experiences.

Of course, the week before you left on vacation, everything at work was insane! Everyone and their mothers were coming to you with complex projects because they all knew you were going to be away for an entire week. After that last day at work, you were in a frenzy getting ready! There was the planning, the packing, who's going to pick up your mail, who will watch Sparky, etc., etc., etc. You were in vacation readiness mode on steroids!

Then it finally arrives, VACATION DAY! You wake up early, you fight traffic on the way to the airport, you find parking, you get everyone into the airport, and then you see the line for Security is 19 miles long and is moving like molasses on a mid-winter day in Detroit. On top of that, your wife keeps giving you "the look" because you were too cheap to do TSA Pre-Check for the whole family.

You finally make it through Security and rush to your gate, you board the plane, find homes for the luggage, get seated in your appropriate seats, and then your six-year-old has to go to the bathroom. You both fight your way to the back of the plane while telling them to hurry up before the flight takes off. You both squeeze yourselves into the phone booth of a bathroom, bump your head on the ceiling and then finally rush back to your seat.

You endure the cramped accommodations of the flight while questioning your sanity. As soon as you land at your destination, you get everyone off the plane. You rush to baggage claim and scan for your luggage. You stand outside to wait with 900 other people for the bus that will take you to your car rental location. Your wife asks why we have to take the bus to a remote rental car location when all of the other "Big name" rental car companies are located at the airport. You mumble under your breath about some special deal and forge onto the bus with your 16 pieces of luggage. You arrive at the Super El Cheapo car rental location that has goats and chickens running around outside. You push your crew to get their luggage off the bus and into the building. Inside it is tiny and cramped, and the temperature is a balmy 86 degrees. The one and only staff person is as motivated as a snail in a race. It takes 2 hours to get your car, and the first question your wife says is, "What is that funky smell?" You mumble about the need for air fresheners, and then begin the navigation battle to find your hotel. Everyone is hot, sweaty, tired, and irritable. Then you proclaim, "Hey kids, aren't we having a great time?!?"

The next morning you get your jet-lagged family up at the crack of dawn and head to the theme park because you want to get your full money's worth out of those overpriced, expensive tickets. You spend the entire day standing in eternally long, hot lines so you can have the thrill of a 2-minute ride. Then, you and the family rush to the next ride to repeat the process. You stay to the bitter end to take in the fireworks. You finally drag everyone out of the park, through the parking lot, pile in the stinky rental car, and head back to the hotel. You repeat the process every day of the trip and then repeat the ride home in just as chaotic fashion as the trip there.

Whenever you finally arrive home, the sheer exhaustion you feel is excruciating. You now *hate* the people you love the most, and you are more stressed-out than before you left. Your wife stares blankly at you and says, "Next year, we are going to sit on a beach somewhere and stare at the waves." Sound familiar?

The goal of a vacation is to relax, not collapse. It should be a time that allows you to leave the stress-filled world behind and spend it in a quiet, restful place, giving you a much-needed change of scenery and allowing your batteries to recharge.

Food for thought:
In the past decade, a new word "staycation "was coined, which is the combination of vacation and stay. The name, Staycation, has become accepted enough to have been added to *Merriam-Webster's Collegiate Dictionary* in 2009. A Staycation is a period when you stay at home and enjoy activities close to your home. Staycations have become very popular for many reasons: financial (you do not have to have lodging elsewhere) as well as not being exhausted after the vacation is over. Still, more importantly, it gives you the time to recharge without the stress that often accompanies vacations.

This can indeed be a way to turn off that unhealthy vacation stress switch!

If you are planning a vacation, do not try to cut corners by saving a few pennies here or there. If you really can't afford the vacation you originally wanted, then choose something you can afford. If what is most affordable are day trips, then think "Staycation."

And, whether it is a vacation or a staycation, do something every year to recharge your batteries. It is better to be blessed than stressed.

CHAPTER TWENTY-TWO
IT ALWAYS COMES OUT IN THE WASH

A note from Rich:

As a teenager, I had a summer job working in a kitchen at an upscale assisted living facility for the elderly in Madison, New Jersey. My fellow dishwasher Sam, who was from Trinidad, once said to me in his great accent, "You know Holmes, my wife washed my brand-new undershirts together with our fiberglass curtains and, Mon, I was itching like crazy!"

Sam and I had some great times together as we scrubbed pots and pans and washed tons of dishes.

The chef had two sets of knives. Every week a knife sharpening service would stop by and pick up the collection that had been used and drop off a sharpened set. These knives were sharp, really sharp. You could rest the blade of the knife on top of a tomato, and it would slice right through it on its own.

I worked at a large double sink that, when I arrived at 11 am, would be full of dirty pots and pans soaking in murky water.

I would dig in and work my way to the bottom. Several times when I was reaching into the dirty water, I grabbed the blade of one of the super-sharp knives. It would have sliced my fingers if they had not been so waterlogged and softer than usual. That prompted me to storm into the kitchen, strongly "informing" everyone NOT to put sharp knives into the sink!

Whatever you put into the wash will always show up when you remove it. Over the years, my family has mistakenly washed pens that leaked ink ruining clothes and chewing gum that stuck to other garments in the dryer. We always had that unfortunate ah-ha moment when we discovered the mess, ever too late to fix it.

Stress is a force in and of itself. Not only will it come out, but it will come out with power. It can manifest itself in many ways, such as anger, bingeing, or even obsessive cleaning.

If you try to stuff it, then it can come out as physical illnesses due to a suppressed immune system.

The only safe approach is not to allow or give power to stress in the first place. That way, you will not have to deal with any unpleasant surprises. This healthier approach is guaranteed to leave a fresh, clean feeling.

CHAPTER TWENTY-THREE

KIDS ARE SPONGES AND HOW TO PROTECT THEM

Deeply concerned parents are sitting in the Principal's office, confronting the fact that their child is apparently a bully. Not just a bully, but also one of the worst bullies the school has ever had.

"How could this happen?" They ask the Principal. They live in a beautiful home in a safe neighborhood; everything their child needs is provided. The Principal asks them, "Do the two of you ever argue?"

The wife says, "All the time. Isn't that normal?" She then gives a sharp glare at her husband and adds, "Especially when you leave your clothes all over the floor! Lazy bum!" The husband snaps back, "Talk about being lazy. I bust my butt at work all day so you can have a maid, but I come home to a microwave dinner!"

The Principal now understands why the child is a bully.

Every word that you speak will either bring forth life or death, blessings, or curses. Children absorb EVERYTHING their parents say. They not only absorb everything, but they are the DNA of their parents. Parents are also the first authority figure a child knows, so they are tuned to their frequency much more than any outsider.

From birth, children trust their parents 100%. The effects of prolonged stress over time wears away at that trust. Unlike the world's view that parents should provide material possessions to their children, the most significant two things a child needs from their parents are trust and love.

If you want your children to grow up into healthy mature adults, then the tone you set in your home is not only crucial; it is foundational. Therefore, we beg you never to fight or belittle each other in front of your children. Never. That is one of the most destructive things you can do. It goes to the core of a child. And it sets the example of how your children should treat their spouses.

For that matter, you should never argue or belittle each other. Period. Most arguments are caused by people's inability to handle stress. The argument is just the vehicle that is used to vent the pressure caused by the stress.

Every word you speak with the wrong tone of voice is causing harm to your children. Whatever stress you transfer to your children, WILL COME OUT in them! You can be assured that you will not like any of the ways that it could manifest itself, such as reckless driving, drinking, drugs, premarital sex, fighting. Just to name a few possibilities.

A personal note from Rich:

I have been in the homes of families where the husband and wife are constantly communicating by yelling at each other. The TV is blaring, and their kids are bouncing off the walls. Only their dog is smart enough to hide. It is brutally unpleasant. The tone you set is so critical to the success of your children. Keep it calm, positive, and stable.

I grew up in the '60s, where smoking was not considered to be as taboo as it is today. Both my parents smoked—my dad a pipe and mom cigarettes. We would be on long car trips, and they would light up without even opening the car window. I can also remember how I used to sit on the arm of my dad's easy chair so he could help me with my homework while he smoked his pipe. Today we would consider that almost a form of child abuse. Back then, the harmful effects of secondhand smoke were practically unknown."

Stress is absorbed in the same way as smoke. Whatever stress you sow into your children will almost always manifest itself in some form later. Even worse is if that stress stays bottled up for years, growing and affecting every relationship they have with anyone.

To Remember

Love is the ONLY four-letter word that needs to be spoken in your home.

More is caught than taught, and if you want your kids to turn out right, then never fight.

If arguing is out, then how do you solve problems in your marriage?

The fact is that MOST of your problems are nowhere as large as they seem and *never* insurmountable. Being stressed out is what makes them seem overwhelming. The number of issues that appear to be problems will decline in direct proportion with the amount of stress you release.

So, if you see yourself in this situation, we strongly encourage you to begin immediately releasing your stress and seek counseling to help relieve the stress.

Once you are free of stress, your children will be able to soak up all the goodness that will then freely pour from you. Your family will be stronger and happier, and you all deserve it!

CHAPTER TWENTY-FOUR

WHERE YOUR "GO-TO" STARTS, MEANS EVERYTHING

You just had an extremely stressful day, and all you want to do is ______________________. (fill in the blank)

That is your "Go-To." It is an immediate action that temporarily relieves the symptoms of stress.

"Go-Tos" vary significantly from one person to the next. The bigger question is, "Where did your Go-To come from?"

Most likely, it was fashioned from your childhood. When your parents were stressed, did they head out to the local ice cream store for a triple dipple, fudge brownie, ice cream, with mountains of whipped cream, laden with sprinkles, and capped with a cherry on top? Did they reach for a bottle to numb the stress? Head to the Mall only to maul their finances and add to debt? When you were a child and came home from a tough day at school, did your mom serve you your favorite comfort food? If so, that very well may be what your "GO-TO" is today.

Can you imagine a family that all chooses to go for a jog after a stressful day instead of an unhealthy choice? One of the most important things parents can do for their children is to model healthy "Go-To" options. This one act can save your children from a lifetime of battling mountains of debt, substance abuse, divorces, health issues, and the list goes on.

The next time you have a stressful day, before you choose a negative "GO-TO," remember how important it is to your children's future success.

If you impart healthy "Go-Tos," you just made a significant step in blessing your child's future.

Even if you display healthy "Go-Tos" and you teach your children how to handle money, take care of their health and to be responsible, hard-working members of society, it can all evaporate ***if they are surrounded by stress***. Even if you raise your child doing everything idealistically, it can all go out the window if their upbringing is surrounded by chaos.

Life is very challenging on its own. Children today experience stresses in their lives that we cannot even fathom. The greatest gift a child can be given is to be shown how to handle stress. If you do everything possible to create a stress-free home, the need for "Go-Tos" is greatly diminished.

Raising your children in a stress-free home is one of the most important things you can do to build a foundation of how life can truly be lived. You can do this!!

CHAPTER TWENTY-FIVE

HOW TO $AVE YOUR MARRIAGE

"Whoever says money can't buy happiness doesn't know where to shop!"

It was a funny bumper sticker that initially made me laugh. However, it got me thinking about "the all mighty dollar." I started thinking about how many people buy things they can't afford to impress people they don't like. I started thinking about how many knock down, drag-out, fights have started over money. I started thinking about how many married couples have legitimate struggles with money.

There is an adage: "money problems are why most marriages fail." On the surface, most people would instantly agree to that being a true statement. Most would agree that every married couple should be required to take a course on money management. However, it is almost entirely false. Money management wouldn't make much of a difference at all in the success of marriages. For decades the U.S. divorce rate has held steady around 50%.

Through the good times and the bad, through financial booms and busts, the rate of marriages that fail has not changed.

So the questions become:
Are half the couples that try marriage that difficult to live with?
Are half of the people who get married mistakenly picking the wrong partner?
Are only half of all adults committed to their marriage vows?

Of course, we are better than that. We are incredibly more competent and more successful than that.

However, every married couple is blindsided by a problem they never saw coming yet knew it was going to hit: Stress.

The real culprit to the money dilemma is the high level of stress that couples are faced with every day. This stress causes a chain reaction that can spiral out of control, causing substantial problems. One of the biggest challenges is the perceived need to spend money on things that give them instant gratification. It is this "Go-To" or a quick fix of instant gratification that only temporarily numbs their stress.

Most couples are made up of two vastly different types of people: the Saver and the $pender. Of course, this is not a problem if they make more than they spend every month, but that is rarely the case.

The Saver's standard answer is to set up a monthly budget. Control the spending. Monitor the dollars and count the cents. Then the constraints of a budget begin to pile up on the $pender. The stress levels of the stressed-out $pender begin to compound because they start feeling confined by the shackles of the spreadsheet. The Saver took away their "Go-To" stress relief, so stress begins to build.

Eventually, the $pender becomes stressed to the point they have to fix the problem the only way they know how, RETAIL THERAPY! They start spending for instant gratification. Binge spending because it is their Go-To, feel-good fix.

However, when the receipts are totaled, the Saver is now the one who is completely stressed! They then need to get their stress fix the only way they know how, by tightening the budget belts yet again. The spiral has begun. The $pender is fighting the Saver; the Saver is challenging the $pender, both forgetting they are on the same team.

REMEMBER: Money problems are just a symptom. Stress is the creepy culprit pulling the strings.

We can prove this point. Even if you doubled each struggling couple's income, they would still have "money" problems. The $pender would increase the amount they stress spend and increase the stress for the $aver to save.

High levels of stress over a prolonged period can even make nice well-grounded people cranky and irritable. This chases the love out the window and starts the door slamming fights. Stress pushes even rational thinking people into the emotional realm where wounded feelings take the place of clear problem-solving.

Stress turns fun-loving couples into individual, self-centered pleasure seekers. If you want to have a successful marriage, then remove the stress and be blessed.

As a relaxed couple, you can now sit back and watch your "money problems" melt away.

CHAPTER TWENTY-SIX

WHAT GOES UP, MUST COME DOWN AND DOWN AND DOWN

Rich's great fall:

The ladder stretched one and a half stories upward to the top of my Connecticut home. Because of its angle, my face was only a few inches away from the soffit that I was aggressively scraping to prepare for new paint. After 20 minutes of this work, I discovered a small hole where the soffit met the shingles. Just as I started to scrape this area, a tiny sparrow flew out of the hole, right in front of my face! I was so startled that I instinctively jumped backward into mid-air! Gravity did its thing, and down I went! When I regained my composure and was standing again, I looked at the ground and saw that my feet left imprints about four inches deep in the Connecticut clay. Thank God that I landed on the very section of ground that I had dug up the previous year to bury a drainpipe. Otherwise, the earth would have been much harder and bruised more than just my pride.

I climbed back up the ladder and finished scrapping the soffit. Feeling accomplished and alive, I went on to play two hard sets of tennis. I felt great! However, the next day it felt like every muscle in my body hurt. Fortunately, it only lasted for a day.

Just like the instinct to jump from a ladder whenever a tiny bird surprises you, people in a stressed state will almost always react rather than respond. The direction they will head is the same as falling from a ladder, straight down.

Stressed people focus on immediate relief, which means some form of instant gratification, otherwise known as their "Go-To." It may be a positive "Go-To" or a negative "Go-To," but stress has tricked you into thinking that you must have it NOW.

Typically our "Go-Tos" are self-indulgent and carnal. Carnal means that it is one of the five senses; those things that you can see, smell, hear, taste, and touch.

Stress will turn a well-grounded person into a "carnal person." That is a self-centered, hedonistic pleasure seeker who only wants immediate gratification for his or her satisfaction.

During stressful situations, this behavior may seem like a "natural" response. But in reality, the stressed person has backed himself or herself into a corner. A corner that has two strong walls on each side, and because of the pressure of stress pushing against them, their vision at that point can only be of survival. That is not a good place to be. It would be the equivalent of a soldier pinned down in a wet, muddy foxhole that has been under vicious attack for days with bombs and bullets flying overhead and then deciding that they need a break from the battle. So, he takes out a picnic basket filled with white table linen, candles, a fresh bouquet in a beautiful glass vase, a delicious spread of food and sets it up right there in the line of fire. It might be a temporarily lovely distraction, but it would only be a matter of time before devastating consequences would occur.

Having a carnal "Go-To" for stress relief is no different. The purpose of your "Go-To" is to relieve the pressure, or else you will reach your breaking point. That is a horrible place to be.

Perhaps one of the most unknown and harmful effects of carnal living is that it shuts off access to your ability to connect spiritually. It's "your way" or the "highway." There is no way to connect spiritually when this self-serving lifestyle has taken control.

For example, have you ever been in your place of worship and trying to engage with the service while you were consumed with stress? Were you able to truly connect? Of course not! There is virtually no possible way to communicate with anyone, spiritually or emotionally, on a genuine level when you have allowed the selfish person – that lives within all of us – to take control.

There is a Cherokee tale of an old Cherokee Indian who was teaching his grandson about life. The sage and wise man said to his grandson, “There is a fight going on inside me. It is a terrible fight, and it is between two wolves. One is evil — He is anger, envy, sorrow, regret, greed, arrogance, self-pity, guilt, resentment, inferiority, lies, false pride, superiority, and ego.”

He continued, “The other is good—He is joy, peace, love, hope, serenity, humility, kindness, benevolence, empathy, generosity, truth, compassion, and faith. The same fight is going on inside of you — and inside every other person, too.”

The grandson thought about it for a minute and then asked his grandfather, “Which wolf will win?”

The old Cherokee replied, “The one you feed.”

This proverb describes how it is when you attempt to only deal with the symptoms of stress. You will inevitably react drastically to the smallest things, like being startled by a sparrow. You will feed a gnawing desire within you in an attempt to pacify a lurking wolf of stress.

Freeing yourself from the grip of stress will allow you to be better prepared to handle anything that life throws at you. It keeps the speed bumps from becoming stop signs, equipping you to respond versus react. It allows you to muzzle the harmful desires you might have and nourish all those that are good.

It is a must if you want to be blessed and not stressed.
We are here to help you!

CHAPTER TWENTY-SEVEN
NEVER WORRY AGAIN

"Worry is like paying a debt you don't owe." –Mark Twain

Worry happens when you are trying to control something you have no control over. It is one of the fastest ways to increase the level of stress in your life. You know the feeling: knot in the belly, the tension in the neck, headache between the eyes. It can control your every thought.

There was a man named Fred who worked for years in a department with twenty other people. He was known as the company "worry-wart." He worried about everything! He worried about the quality of his work. He worried about his job security. He worried about his personal life. He worried about his family and his children and his car and his bills. He even worried about other people's problems. He was consumed with worry. Because of his worrywart attitude, he was a drain to be around.

However, one day Fred came into work whistling a happy tune. His co-workers immediately noticed a change in his entire demeanor. He went through the whole day and did not worry about anything. Finally, all his co-workers just had to ask what had caused this dramatic and extreme change. They wanted to know why he was not worrying anymore.

Joe said, "Fred, we all know that you worry all the time, and today has been different. What have you done differently to keep you from worrying?" Fred replied, "It was the easiest thing I've ever done. I hired a professional worrier to worry for me."

Somewhat astonished, Joe replied, "Wow! That is great, and it seems to work for you. By the way, how much does this professional worrier cost?" Fred calmly replied, "$500 a day."

Shocked, Joe said, "$500 a day! How are you going to afford to pay him?" Fred said, "I don't care; that's his problem."

A humorous story, but the point comes down to the fact that the majority of the time, you could decide not to be a worrywart. Realistically, the majority of the things you worry about don't even happen! Someone once said, "I have 99 problems, and 86 of them are completely made up scenarios in my head that I'm stressing about for absolutely no logical reason."
Does that hit close to home?

Worry never got anyone anything except more wrinkles. So, "Don't worry. Be happy!"

CHAPTER TWENTY-EIGHT
THE STRESS FREE DIET

"I am trying to do everything I am supposed to do to lose weight, but it isn't coming off." That is what my frustrated co-worker Desiree said to me. She is like millions if not billions of people who have: Cut calories, go for long boring walks on treadmills, cut out sweets, carbs, fat, processed foods, meat, dairy, and are only left with air to eat. They have gone Vegan, practice mediation, starve themselves. Almost all of them losing the battle of the bulge.

They walk around hungry, which makes them crabby hangry people. They have tried countless food diets only to fail again.

Since you are reading this book, you know what I am going to offer up as the dirty rotten culprit that is causing all this weight gain.

Yes, it is stress.

But, there are two parts to the equation.

1. We have discussed that when people are stressed, they resort to their Go-To for instant gratification. They will often consume unhealthy foods that can certainly add to weight gain.

But what if they have strong willpower and are denying themselves the unhealthy foods? Why are they still having trouble shedding the pounds?

2. Secret revealed. Let me introduce you to our friend called Cortisol. When people are stressed, they are in Fight, Flight, or Freeze

response, Cortisol levels in their body rise. It floods their body with the glucose that gives immediate energy for their large muscles. Cortisol is like rocket fuel. If you don't fight the tiger or run away from it (both intensive exercise activities), it will stay unused. If you are only stressed once or twice throughout life, then it is not a problem. But when people are in an almost constant state of stress, then there is a lot of stored rocket fuel (Cortisol), which is a fat-storing hormone.

The best way to burn that stored rocket fuel is to do intensive exercises. A lot of people are not in the proper shape to safely do that kind of workout. Even if they wanted to, they should be checked out by their doctor first.

That is in a nearly perfect world. The fact is that when most people come home from a stressful day, they barely have enough energy to make it back. Let alone go for an intensive workout. They are drained and exhausted.

A note from Rich:

I worked for the first four months at the New York Times as an Associate Art Director. That meant that the current Art Director was my boss, and he handed me one project at a time to complete. Then he left, and they promoted me to Art Director. And the proverbial peanut butter hit the fan. I was no longer able to sit in my corner quietly, working on a project. I had a constant stream of department heads bringing in one project after another. It was like they all came out of the woodwork. Talk about a stressful day. I dragged myself to my car and drove home. My wife asked me how your first day was? I think I said I was going to lie down for a while, which turned into more than a while.

How are we supposed to burn the stored Cortisol if we are exhausted?

You can't. But you can control your situation so that you will not be in a constant state of stress. By turning off your Stress Switches (Chapter 8), you will be lowering your day-to-day stress load, keeping you from increasing Cortisol in your body. So if you encounter a single stressful event, your levels should return to normal very quickly.

That is the secret why most people gain or cannot lose weight.

CHAPTER TWENTY-NINE

IN A HURRY TO GO NOWHERE

The plane touches down and makes its way to the terminal gate.

Over the airplane intercom, "Ladies and Gentlemen, please remain in your seats with your seatbelts fastened until the plane comes to a complete stop and the captain turns off the seatbelt sign."

As the plane is about to stop, everyone grabs their seat belts in anxious anticipation of the captain hitting that button that sends out the chime and turns off the seat belt sign. Everyone impatiently waits and stares at the illuminated seat belt light above each seat.

The flight attendant comes back over the intercom and warns those rebels, which everyone heard release their seat belts early, to keep it fastened until the captain turns off the sign.

The seat belt light remains illuminated. People are chomping at the bit as their fingers tap on the seat belt clasp as if to be preparing for a lightning-fast quick draw release.

Then it happens. The moment that has been waited for with anxious aggravation and anticipation! The chime rings! The seat belt light goes off! The race is on! Seat belts fly off! People leap from their seats, grabbing their bags out of the overhead bins with lightning speed and precision! The aisle of the plane is instantly jam-packed with people from the aisle seats, who are now cramming together, and people from the inner seats behind them are pressing forward to get out into the aisle before anyone from a row behind them gets out.

However, no one moves. Like cold maple syrup being poured on a blustery winter day, the jet bridge begins to move painstakingly slowly towards the plane's door.

Every passenger frustratingly waits to be released yet again. Stress levels spike over things entirely out of their control. They were in a hurry to go nowhere fast.

Similar to the people who cannot seem to wait for any event to end. They start heading to the door like they are being pulled out with the tide in the ocean. They do not stay around and engage with anyone; they go. If someone were to ask them why they were in such a hurry, they would likely reply, "We just have to go."

"They" are the people who have lived a life of always being on the go. So naturally, when something is over, it is just time to go. Maybe this is you – the person who is always on the go, or perhaps you know someone who is the "goer."

This lifestyle makes it hard to develop friends and build quality relationships. Some may wonder why they don't have many friends. This "we just have to go" lifestyle can rob the joy out of an otherwise entirely fantastic event. It is a stress switch that they have turned on for absolutely no reason.

What would happen if you filled the gas tank of your car, put the car in neutral, and then pressed the gas pedal to the floor, revving the engine at full throttle until it ran out of gas? Once you burned all the fuel in the tank, you then fill it with gas again and repeated the process?

Eventually, the engine would crater! Your car's engine was not designed to run in this matter, and an eventual breakdown is inevitable.

In the same manner, you were never designed to run continuously at full speed, or maybe we should say “fool speed.” Eventually, that stress will have some adverse effects on your body, your engine. Remember, the word “recreation” actually means the opportunity to recreate yourself.

Just as the designers of the roads did not install guardrails to protect the trees and bushes, guardrails were set up to be warning signs and to protect you. But you must pay attention to precautions on both the road you are on and to the way you are driving. We live in a world that has pre-conditioned us all to believe that we have to operate at record-breaking speeds. This same precautionary mindset should be applied to your stress switches.

A note from Matt:

I have always loved to work. For years my motto was, ‘There’s only “go” not any “whoa”.’ After spending several weeks of working every day while only stopping for church on Sunday morning, my sweet wife Katy said, ‘You do realize that after He created the world even God took a day off.’ That thought resonated with me to my core. I realized that I was running at “fool speed”, and I had to take time to refuel my tank so that I could run at full speed when full speed was needed.

Thoughts to remember

If you are continuously in a stressed-out state, then maybe it is time to take your foot off the gas, apply the brakes, and find something that will fuel your soul.

This action is often the only way that you will ever be able to arrive at the scenic outlook that gives you the view of your life’s real purpose.

Going somewhere with purpose is better than going nowhere fast.

CHAPTER THIRTY

HOW TO GO BACK TO SLEEP IN THE MIDDLE OF THE NIGHT

You are fast asleep dreaming of lying on a beautiful beach without a care in the world. Suddenly, you are wide awake. You have no clue what disrupted your peaceful slumber. Maybe, you heard something, or perhaps it was the weather outside or a family member coughing, or maybe it was a trip to the bathroom that woke you up. You look at the clock and discover that it is only 2:00 am.

Regardless, you want and desperately need to go back to sleep immediately. You set your alarm clock to go off at 6:30. You've got to get back to sleep as soon as possible! However, instead of falling back into your peaceful slumber, you stare at the ceiling.

You can hear the ticking of the clock as seconds march slowly by. 2:30AM, 3:00AM, 3:30AM. Nothing.

You NEED sleep, and you NEED to get back to it immediately. Yet here you are, staring at the ceiling—your mind races from one random thing to another.

4:00 AM, 4:30 AM, more time passes. You toss, and you turn, and your frustration grows.

You focus on the things you HAVE to accomplish throughout your day, which only adds to your insomnia. How are you going to achieve it if you don't have a good night's sleep? There is absolutely no way that it's going to be possible, much less enjoyable! Now you are adding stress to insomnia, and you want to sleep.

You are now desperate. In a last-ditch effort, you start counting sheep. After you get to 39, you remember that you don't even like sheep, and you become even more frustrated and stressed.

You grab your phone to try and pass the time, but that does nothing, so you put it back down. Mr. Sandman has left the building!

Has this ever happened to you? Chances are it has, because it happens to almost everyone. Take comfort. There is a method that can help you overcome it and get the sleep you need.

It works similar to your Go-Tos when you are stressed, but in this case, you direct it differently. It is called "Going to your Happy Place." I know that sounds silly, but try it next time you can't sleep.

Your Happy Place is the real or imaginary place that shows up in your daydreams. If you love to go camping, then start daydreaming at night about setting up your tent, next to a beautiful stream in the shadows of a stunning view — the warm glow from your campfire illuminating your loved one's face. Just let your imagination take you there with every detail imaginable. Of course, since you control the dream, you can feel the perfect temperature, you can see your ideal scene, smell the sweetest of aromas, and you can hear the ideal sounds. Peace and tranquility abound.

Focusing on your Happy Place will quiet your mind, relax your body, and allow your daydream to transition into a night dream.

I practice this most nights when I get in bed, and I am asleep in a matter of moments. Another benefit is that it sets the direction of my dreams. I am starting at my Happy Place, and not the problems I encountered that day.

What better way to ease into slumber land than by starting where everything is wonderful! And, as the old song says, "...you can be sure that if you're feeling right, a daydream will last long into the night..."

Welcome home, Mr. Sandman. We've been expecting you. Enjoy your ZZZ's.

CHAPTER THIRTY-ONE

YOU HAVE SOME NERVE

When we defined stress and its effects, we talked at length about the central nervous system and how it is what controls everything about you. The fact is, you do have some nerve!

Within your central nervous system is the Vagus Nerve. The Vagus Nerve is like your body's Amazon River, wandering throughout the body while sending messages from your brain to your vital organs and countless other places. It is so named because it "wanders" like a vagabond. This is the nerve that controls your parasympathetic nervous system, the source of your rest, digest, and repair. It is responsible for overseeing a vast range of crucial functions, but one of its primary functions is to tell your body how to respond to stress.

Scared Stressed!

A Note from Rich when he was scared stressed:

I remember as a 12-year-old riding my bike past the firehouse in New Jersey. Everything was splendid until a deafening fire horn began blaring! In a split second, my mind transitioned from Rest, Digest, and Restore mode to Fight, Flight, or Freeze mode. That sudden sound caused a wave of pins and needles to travel from my head to my toes. Fortunately, it only lasted a few seconds, but it did freak me out. My Vagus Nerve was scared!

A Note from Matt when he was scared stressed:

On a business trip to Minneapolis, Minnesota, I remember resting comfortably in bed on the 14th floor of my hotel. Suddenly, an ear-piercing alarm went off, and a man's voice came over a loudspeaker stating, "There is a fire on the 14th floor! Please exit your rooms immediately and proceed to the nearest stairwell to exit the building!" I was startled to my feet! I quickly exited my room and found that smoke was filling the hall! I assure you, there was no more "Rest, Digest, and Restore" to be had! Shortly after that, the culprit was discovered as someone who set their trash can on fire with a discarded, illegally lit cigarette. It was a frightening situation for my Vagus Nerve.

Those are two prominent examples of the Vagus Nerve, triggering the need for a rapid response! However, sometimes it can be much less noticeable. For example, have you ever had a stressful or strenuous day at work? If your job keeps you in Fight, Flight, or Freeze mode, how can you transition yourself to Rest, Digest, and Repair mode? That is a less obvious example of the Vagus Nerve trigger.

And relaxed to a stop

The Vagus Nerve also has incredible power to relax you to a stop as well.

The Vagus Nerve can:

1. Prevent inflammation throughout your body. This new field is known as bioelectronics, which may be the future of medicine.

2. It helps you make memories that you remember.

3. It helps you breathe without even thinking about it.

4. It acts like the heart's natural pacemaker.

5. It turns on the Rest, Digest and Restore response.

6. It is like a walkie-talkie between your gut and brain.

Note from Rich:

Several times when I have gone for minor surgery, and I have had a Vasovagal Syncope response. It causes a sudden drop in blood pressure sending a wave from my head to my stomach of feeling faint, clammy, and profusely sweating. This has happened with as little stimulus as watching a nurse start an IV in my hand. The medical staff lays me back, and my symptoms are relieved rather quickly. The overstimulation of the vagus nerve caused that reaction.

Vagus Nerve in training

There are several hacks you can do to stimulate your Vagus Nerve, which in turn, will calm you.

- One of the first, and easiest, is to try taking deep breaths and exhaling completely, or say a calm, thoughtful prayer, or even try meditating to calm your mind and settle the nerve.

- Because the Vagus Nerve runs through your mouth, you can also sing at the top of your lungs, or hum, or laugh to stimulate the nerve. All of which can help inform your Vagus Nerve that it is okay to settle down. Gargling with water can also help stimulate the Vagus Nerve.

- Positive relationships with friends and animals can be helpful.

- Eating more healthy fiber and keeping your gut health in excellent condition is even another form that can be beneficial.

There are exciting breakthroughs on the horizon with all the new and upcoming research into the power this nerve has to impact your ability to control stress positively. However, the ultimate goal is to take charge of your emotions and get your nerves under control.

The next time you feel your Vagus Nerve has taken a "Vegas vacation," try some or all of these tips to see what will help you calm your nerve most effectively.

CHAPTER THIRTY-TWO
HOW TO AVOID THE EMOTION COMMOTION

It was in the predawn hours before the sun came up. I swiped my credit card at the gas station and reached for the gas pump to fill up my car. Inadvertently, I grabbed the diesel pump by mistake. Fortunately for me and my car, I caught myself just before I made a grave mistake. You cannot put diesel fuel into a vehicle that runs on gasoline. You will immediately have all kinds of problems.

Unlike your car, your brain was actually designed to run on two mental "fuels." One is rational fuel, and the other is emotional fuel.

Your body was designed to run on rational fuel 95% of the time. Rational thinking allows you to make the decisions that are by far in your best interest. They are the logical thoughts and decisions that are based on facts and realities. It is this process that allows you to balance your thoughts, consider others, and arrive at acceptable and logical decisions.

Emotional thinking is best described as feelings like love, compassion, joy, and peace of mind. It can also fuel emotions like hate, resentment, anger, fear. Emotions are those tricky things in your brain that can cause you to think of all kinds of thoughts, good and bad. They can pull you to glorious mountaintops or drag you into dark valleys. When emotional thinking is dominant in your daily existence, your moods can fluctuate radically like a rollercoaster. Many times, you might even try to gratify or squelch your emotions with negative or positive "Go-Tos."

How you eat is a great example. People who run on rational thinking will order a healthy option because it is what their body needs. An emotional thinking person will order whatever satisfies a craving, but with only temporary results.

The biggest problem is when you add stress to your life, it can keep you mired in emotional thinking and influence you to make poor decisions consistently. Remember, emotions will triumph over facts every time. You can have all the facts, figures, data, and proof that what you are doing is good, necessary, and right; however, all of that may go out the window if your emotions are involved. Emotional thinking is far more powerful than rational thinking.

A personal story from Rich:
Living in Tampa, Florida we had Hurricane Irma make a beeline for our city. For days the track from the national hurricane center had the line going over our house. Even though Floridians are supposed to prepare, they rarely do. People were running around in sheer panic mode. For some strange reason, Floridians only stock up on water right before a hurricane. Our neighbor waited in line at Costco for a case of water only to have it stolen inside the store when she briefly turned her back.

People were in panic mode, buying all kinds of stuff they usually did not purchase. Even though Hurricane Irma was a unique weather event, many people live an emotional lifestyle every day. Eventually, this Emotional Thinking will become the new normal, and they could spend the rest of their lives feeding their ever so needy emotions instead of making sound rational decisions that are in their best interest.

Full-time emotional thinking is incompatible with the way we are designed to live and should be a warning sign that stress levels need to be significantly reduced. However, this may not be evident to the emotional thinker, so a trusted friend or loved one may need to point this out gently. If you are the trusted friend or loved one, be mindful that emotions overrule facts almost every time, so you should handle this gently with love and respect.

CHAPTER THIRTY-THREE
ENJOYING YOUR STRESS-FREE LIFE

The traffic light turns red just as you approach it. You respond with, "Yes! I get to wait at the light. It will give me a few moments to relax from driving."

You arrive at the grocery and find the few items you need quickly. As you head to check out, you spot an open lane. Just as you turn your cart in that direction, another person with a fully loaded cart shows up. You allow them to go in front of you even though it will add 10 minutes to your time in the store. You think to yourself, "Yes! I get to bless them."

You are in the crowded waiting room at the doctor's office, and another person walks in. You immediately get up and give them your seat. "Yes! I get to stand, and I get to bless them."

You go to get a cup of coffee at work, and you notice there is only one cup left in the pot. You fill your cup and take the time to make a fresh pot. "Yes! Better to bless than stress."

You are at a restaurant, and after ordering your food, it is taking an eternity to arrive. You are glad because you can spend more time staring into your soulmate's eyes sitting across from you. Besides, who needs food when you are in love? Or, you are at the same restaurant by yourself, so you use the extra time to send text messages to whoever comes to mind just to let them know that you are thinking about them and you care.

You are chilled and relaxed every day. Like everyone, you have a job, family, and responsibilities, but now you only care about what is important to you. You can minimize all the meaningless stuff that monopolizes the majority of the minds of the millions.

You feel a calmness and a peace that you have never had before. It is almost like you are having an out of body experience as you watch everyone else around you who are freaking out from all their stress. You pity their situation because that used to be you, but no longer. You feel like you have been freed from all the stress-producing chaos, and you couldn't be more thankful.

Because of your freedom, when everyone else sees the "storm", you see answers. A stressed mind is confused and uncertain. A stressed mind can be vulnerable to all kinds of poor decisions. Stressed people are, by nature, self-centered people. Calm people, by choice, can bless others.

While hanging out with your friends, you notice almost all they talk about are their problems. Yes, you USED to do the same. Now, you only care about enjoying the time you spend together. You mention something positive, and they all turn and look at you like you said something offensive.

You now have a longing to delve into being a more spiritual person, which can open up a whole new area to explore. It was like stress blocked you from ever going there.

The Bible says, "The peace of God will transcend all understanding."

You are no longer drawn to engage in the same types of entertainment you once thought you enjoyed. Shows or movies with drama that you used to watch no longer appeal to you. The modern media almost repulse you, so you keep it turned off. You start to appreciate classical music, soft jazz, or spiritual music in place of the stressful headbanging music you used to listen to.

You have rediscovered the glory of nature. You love strolling through parks and viewing anything full of life. You can now hear the birds singing amid the craziness. You can see beauty all around you, where you once saw nothing. You can find something beautiful in any situation.

You now realize that time is a very precious commodity. You are no longer willing to waste it "being entertained" by other people's twisted thoughts. You recognize that watching entertainment is just viewing and absorbing someone else's imagination. By turning it off, you have turned on one of your most beautiful and powerful assets, YOUR imagination.

You now take the time to ponder and even daydream. Like a horse with blinders, you used to have tunnel vision and only view what was directly in front of you. This new life breaks open your creativity and critical thinking skills.

You feel 20 years younger; the aches and pains seem to have vanished along with the pain in your stressed-out stomach.

Your day is no longer sprinting from one meaningless task to another. It is like you are gliding through each day as if you were walking on air.

Because you are learning to free yourself of stress, you enjoy life more. This new lifestyle is how we were designed to live, a life filled with love, joy, peace, and a sound mind.

If this does not describe your current experiences, then with the help of this book, you are heading out of the darkness and into the stress-free light. You were designed for this. You deserve it. You can do it.

CHAPTER THIRTY-FOUR

RICH'S POSITIVE SIDE OF NEGATIVE SPACE

Have you ever noticed the arrow in the FedEx logo? It is made up of negative space between the "E" and the "X." Negative space is the area around the primary object. For example, a picture on a wall is a positive space; the blank wall is the negative space.

As a graphic designer, I have had clients tell me there is too much "white space" in my design and that I needed to cram in more selling copy. This only makes the design busy and ineffective because people's eyes will not know where to look.

The human mind also operates with positive and negative space. The things you focus on are your positive space, and the items in your background are your negative space. Your imagination operates almost exclusively in your negative space. This includes your creativity and even your hopes.

Stress will put people into fight or flight mode, which slams them into 100% positive space. Instead of the focus being work, spending time with family or friends, or leisurely drives in your car, it is all on stress. The stress completely dissolves your ability to imagine. Your imagination is what gives you hope for today and tomorrow. It's what gets you out of bed each morning.

Stressed people are so wiped out that they often tune into the entertainment world for their imagination, which may not line up with their actual beliefs. They can end up viewing hour after hour of lying, cheating, stealing, murder, sex, drugs, and knocking on the wrong doors. Their imagination has been replaced, and advertisements become more appealing because they have reprogrammed their mind.

Thus, these stressed people end up participating in their "cycle" of stress and duress instead of turning the stress switches off.

I have made a conscious effort to no longer live a stressed life. One of the many benefits is I now spend much more time in my negative space. This mind shift has exploded my creativity and given me enormous amounts of hope. It is almost impossible for me to feel bummed out or have even a bad moment.

How Do I Personally Do This?

To supercharge my negative space, I fast from food for 24 hours every Friday night to Saturday night. It puts me in a relaxed state that propels me into negative space. Amazingly, I look forward to fasting on Saturdays because of the more in-depth time I can spend in my negative space. I have to admit that I also fast for spiritual reasons, not to deprive myself but to enhance my relationship with God. My most intimate and personal exchanges with God come on Saturdays.

As you discover ways to lower your stress, you will find yourself benefiting from the positive side of negative space.

CHAPTER THIRTY-FIVE
POST TRAUMATIC STRESS RELIEVED

Caution: Heavy Chapter Ahead

One of the most misunderstood, yet most dangerous types of stress in existence today is Post-Traumatic Stress Disorder, commonly referred to as PTSD. That being said, this is an extremely heavy chapter. We will share with you a couple of personal stories that have caused us to experience PTSD firsthand. If the stories are too personal or cause you to relive your own stress, we encourage you to skip them and move ahead to the steps of overcoming your situation. Regardless, be of good cheer. There is hope. There is a way to deal with significant stress moments so that you, too, can become the best version of Stress-Free You possible!

A note from Matt:

Saturday, August 3, 11:46 PM is a day that I will not soon forget.

As the self-proclaimed "Gooder Guy," I believe my purpose is to help others to do more, be more, and have more than they ever thought possible. Through speaking engagements and seminars, I LOVE to help others see that life is good, and together we can make it goodER! This past year my career has taken off, and I have been blessed with an abundance of speaking opportunities.

However, this past July came to a close with me only being home for a total of eight days. It was a wonderful and grueling travel schedule that I was blessed to have. The last few days of the month and the first three days of August were a whirlwind. I conducted a four-day training in Louisiana, helped close out a youth training in Dallas, Texas, on Saturday morning August 3, and then that night conducted a keynote at a banquet for the "Live Like Johnny Foundation" just north of Fort Worth, Texas.

Facing a five-hour drive home after the banquet, I told my wife, Katy, that I was just too exhausted to drive that far, that late at night. She completely understood. My wife is a wedding and event planner and very often works late into the night on weekends.

That Saturday, she coordinated a wedding that finished before midnight. I had just made it to my hotel room when she left the wedding venue to head home. As she pulled out onto the road, she called me to tell me about the events of the wedding. According to our phones, we had only been talking for two minutes whenever I heard her scream; the airbags deploy, and then the phone disconnected. A lady who chose to drive drunk blew through a stop sign causing Katy to crash into them.

I have never known sheer panic until that moment. My mind instantly took me to the worst place possible; the fact that she could be dead. Praise God; she was not! Because her phone was connected to her car Bluetooth and the car was now dead, she could not call me. Though hurt and shaken, she had the frame of mind to send me the following four texts:

"My phone won't work."
"I'm okay."
"I got into a wreck."
"Airbags."

I've never been so relieved to receive a text message in all of my life! Although Katy was bruised and suffered a severe concussion, she was alive. Knowing sleep was no longer an option for me. I grabbed my bag and immediately started the arduous drive home. I had to get to where she was. I had to hold her. I had to be with her.

The next few weeks were a struggle, but we were grateful that she was beginning the healing process. However, internally I began to experience a personal shift in the way I felt about my wife. I could feel myself becoming more distant from her and drawing away from her. Multiple times Katy asked me if I was okay, and each time the answer was, "Of course. I'm fine." Internally, I knew I was not. I finally told Katy that I thought I needed to talk to our friend, Beth, who is an incredible counselor, about the wreck because I could tell I was not handling it well.

At our first visit, Counselor Beth put me at ease, and we began to have a genuine conversation about the wreck. She told me about trauma and how it can affect us – all of which was very real to me at that moment. Then she made a statement that I won't soon forget. She said, "At least yours and Katy's relationship is strong. That will help you both get through this." The words I said still haunt me, "That is the problem. I can tell I am pushing her away."

Shocked, but grateful for my confession, Counselor Beth began to ask me a series of questions. She asked how I was pushing Katy away. I said, "By putting a wall around my heart." She asked why I wanted to do that, and I replied with, "Because the wall will protect me from getting hurt again."

Beth countered with, "What is the emotional consequence of having a wall around your heart, and what would that wall eventually do to yours and Katy's relationship?" After a thoughtful pause, I had to admit that my perceived wall of protection would do nothing more than hurt me. Counselor Beth then told me I had to dispute this misconceived untruth that I was trying to convince myself of with real truth. I realized then that I had to ask for help and start tearing down the wall. I had to remove that which was untrue and fill myself with the actual gift I had been given with the blessing of my wife.

As Beth's and my conversation proceeded, she asked additional questions about my past. One of the questions she asked was if I ever had a traumatic or near-death experience. I told her, as a matter of fact, I have an entire speech about it! On January 19, 2015, I had an accident on the farm where I fell and was impaled by a piece of metal in my leg. It came within one inch of hitting my femoral artery. I even titled the speech, "The Power of an Inch."

Beth listened to my story, finished her evaluation, and then gave me a diagnosis that I instantly rejected. She said, "You have every symptom of Post-Traumatic Stress Disorder." I said, "Yeah, right! That's only for warriors and people in the military."

She said, "Unfortunately, that's what most people think."

Throughout that conversation and subsequent others, I learned about "free-floating anxiety" and that when you have a near-death experience or an extremely traumatic situation, your mind commits the entire occurrence to the cellular level. Then at some point, it is possible for another experience or a sound or smell or color to bring it all together and place it in the forefront of your mind. It is almost as if it is still happening. Anything that existed at the time of the stress once experienced again can switch it on in the present as if it is happening in real-time.

This is why it is called POST-traumatic stress.

A Note from Matt's wife, Katy:

There are events and things that will happen in life that will change you. These shocking moments will affect you in a way you cannot predict, plan for, or sometimes even know how to handle. They can also create physical symptoms and times of Post-Traumatic Stress that you must face and deal with to heal completely. In my life, I have experienced some of these moments, one being the car accident that Matt references in the commentary above, but the one I want to share with you occurred in 2013.

Let me first share a little background information so my story will best be understood.

Growing up in Fort Worth, TX, there were three of us that were inseparable from age six to senior year of high school: Kate, Christina, and myself. From slumber parties to birthdays, to summer camp, to prom, college searching, and graduation – we did it all together. Kate got married when we were only 20, and I remember her wedding night like it was a year ago. Christina and I were Kate's Co-Maids of Honor. On her wedding night, we got to stay in the honeymoon suite at the hotel where the wedding was held, because the bride and groom were gifted a fabulous suite in a different hotel and chose to stay there. Christina and I laughed all night, ate the steak dinner that had been brought up for the married couple, and talked about our weddings one day. We planned it all out even though neither of us was anywhere near that moment!

Christina and I went to college only 3 hours away from each other, so we visited one another often and would always have the grandest adventures. Christina was bold, passionate, creative, and fearless. She had a unique ability to turn any situation into a party and made every person feel special. After college, I moved back to Fort Worth, and Christina to California to pursue graduate school. We kept in touch and got together every chance we could! In May of 2010, Christina married the love of her life at a lighthouse in California overlooking the ocean. It was a time so filled with love, and I am thankful that I am now finally able to look back at it without being crushed. Christina and her husband Jacob moved back to Fort Worth after they were married, which I was thrilled about because I got to see them more!

This is an EXTREMELY short and concise sharing of our relationship, but I wanted to try to give you an idea of how close we were and what she means to me. Christina and I had the type of friendship where we could finish each other's sentences, and she knew what I was thinking without me having to say a thing.

Tragically, in April of 2013, Christina had to have surgery because a tumor was found in her brain. I remember sitting at the hospital that day with Kate, waiting for the operation to be over, and to hear the words, "She is okay. It all went well." When we finally got word that she was in recovery and the surgery was over, we were told that the tumor was stage four melanoma. But even though the tumor was cancerous, they said to us that the surgeons were able to get it all. My immediate reaction was a relief. She was going to be okay. They had caught it early enough, and she was going to be just fine.

During her healing process, I spent a lot of time with her. Her husband Jacob is a singer/songwriter/musician, and because noises were very jarring to her healing brain, we would spend time together while Jacob played shows around town. I cherished it and LOVED having this time with her. Because of Christina's progress, in May, we went to this fabulous Italian restaurant in Dallas and celebrated her 27th birthday. It was a magical evening!

Unfortunately, in June, while my family and I were on vacation at the lake, we received some news that crushed me. Christina was back in the hospital because she was having some issues that the doctor believed could either be something new or the remaining effects from her earlier surgery. I did not feel good about it either way and cut my trip short to get back to Texas and be with her.

When I arrived at the hospital two days later, Christina was having hallucinations and had several shunts placed in her brain to try and help alleviate pressure. It was difficult to see her struggling with pain and being attached to machines. Over the next seven weeks, I walked through hell on earth. Christina had a series of surgeries, resulting in the news that her melanoma was back with a vengeance, and that it looked, unlike any other case the surgeon had seen. After two full days of surgeries, and the successful extraction of a cancerous blockage in the 4th ventricle of her brain, we were once again hopeful. Jacob allowed me to sleep in her hospital room after surgery and watch over her so he could try to get some rest. If I remember correctly, I don't think he had slept in about three days. That night after surgery, the nurses and doctor came in every hour on the hour to do cognitive testing and see if she would respond to their voices and prompts. I understand the need for this and the importance of it, but to an already traumatized and hurting young woman, it was quite jarring. After that night, I spent most days, nights, mornings, and weekends when I was not working at the hospital. I missed so much work, but I did not even care. I remember someone asking me back then, "What if they fire you?" That was not as important to me as being with my best friend when she was fighting to live.

The medical team tried radiation to see if it would help kill the melanoma. Still, the cancer came back even more aggressively against the radiation and continued to ravage all of her earthly body. After the unsuccessful radiation treatments ended in mid-July, Christina was moved to a room out of ICU and began hospice care. I sang to her, painted her fingernails her favorite mint green, told her stories, called Kate, and put her on speakerphone so she could talk to Christina. I spent all the time with her that I could. She couldn't speak back to me, and most of the time, at this point, her eyes were closed, but occasionally she would squeeze my hand and hold it for several seconds, letting me know she loved me and was happy I was by her side. Words cannot even begin to describe to you how painful and difficult this journey was to go through and still is to even recall. I saw things I never thought I would see, heard things I wish I could unhear, and put my body under a significant amount of stress and neglect. Looking back, I would not change a single thing about any of it. I was honored to be by her side during this time, and I would do it all over again; I just mean to say it was not easy.

Christina died on August 18, 2013. Something I did not think about during our time in the hospital at all was, what it would be like after she left us. I felt such an indescribable void and sadness. In addition to our grief, we also had to move out. Staying up there for over a month, we had all brought plenty of personal belongings up there during our stay, and we had to move them out in the middle of the night so they could move her and get the room ready for another patient. I got home at about 5:00 AM Sunday the 18th, and I remember just sitting down on the floor in my room and falling apart. I did not come out of my room for a couple of days because I just did not care. I did not have the energy, the desire, or the drive.

I was broken and hurting. I had not cried during much of her time in the hospital, but during her funeral, I could not catch my breath due to how hard I was crying. It was a beautiful service, but I barely remember who we spoke to or saw. She was loved and an inspiration to so many people – there were over 400 people present.

After her service, as I began to come out of my fog, I realized I needed help. I had no idea how to navigate grief like this or how even to begin a healing type journey. I started with a grief share group counseling program at a local church, which helped a lot, but I still struggled after the program was complete. Even years later, I still struggled.

After Matt and I first got married, I was going through my things looking for something, and my hand rested on her mint nail polish that I had used to paint her nails in the hospital. I immediately LOST it and could not breathe. I felt like ocean waves had knocked me over, and I was falling. How could something so small have such a huge physical impact on me three years after losing her? Grief was still playing a part in my journey, but I believe that at this point, I was truly struggling with Post Traumatic Stress. I had worked to deal with my emotions of grief directly after her death, but then I still struggled, and I didn't know what to do. I thought time would heal, and it would get easier. It would eventually go away.

It was not until 2018, five years after Christina had died that I spoke to Counselor Beth, and she identified that I was still experiencing what she thought to be post-traumatic stress. Not simply from her death and from the loss of my dear friend, but from the way in which we lost her. The experience of walking by her side as we were slowly losing her was very traumatic. I learned that in order to move past the trauma aspect of what I had experienced, I had to address it head-on. I had to work through it step by step.

I share all of this with you to reinforce that Post-Traumatic stress can be deeply tied to grief. It can look like grief, and you may not identify at first that it is indeed an additional layer that will require additional work to get through. If you are experiencing anything like this, I want you to know that you are not alone and that there is hope to get through and to the other side.

With the impact, magnitude, and depth that stress can have on our lives, there is a looming question. How then can you deal with major stress?

If you feel that you experience any form of PTSD, please get help from a person trained in dealing with traumatic stress.

In the meantime, here are a few steps you can take to begin the process.

Step One: Realize and accept that you have traumatic stress.

Once we take the time to accept the feeling, we can begin to trace it back to the switch that caused the stress. It may be as simple as accepting the fact that God did not make us have generalized anxiety. That is not normal; it is a switch that has been turned on. When you can realize and accept the moments your body is not being relaxed, you can then begin to figure out the cause. Pay attention to your anxiety. There is always a physical reaction to it—something like your heart racing, profuse sweating, nervous tension, upset stomach, etc. Then you can proceed to step number two.

Step Two: What thoughts are you having during these moments?

When something triggers traumatic stress, your mind goes straight back to the moment. So, ask yourself what was happening around you that caused the flashback. Was it the sound of popcorn popping? Was it a certain aroma? Did you see a color that reminded you of a person? Did something happen to someone else, and it caused you to go back there in your mind? Whenever that happens, you can identify it as a traumatic trigger and start working through it. You can say to yourself, "I do not want to have this reaction to this smell, color, etc. I will work step by step to change this reaction." Take a few deep breaths and try to clear your mind.

Step Three: Create your ideal way to handle the stress when it comes.

For example, whatever it is that puts you in the traumatic spot, say to yourself, "I will ground myself in the now." Maybe say, "That is the past. I am in the present. I am safe. I am grounded in the present."

When you have a flashback, ground yourself in the present. Again, take a breath. Bring your mind into the now. PTSD is trying to tell you that the same thing is happening again, so come up with a solution to do in case it does happen again. Then you are prepared. Know what to do and make a plan to be safe.

Step Four: Take the time to write an essay.

You have to take the time to write the story down of whatever happened to you. Give as many details as you can come up with. Relive the incident word by word. For some of you, this will be incredibly difficult. It may cause you to be anxious, bring to light feelings you thought were buried, and it will be excruciatingly hard. You must do this. Then, you are to read that story out loud, every day, until it no longer bothers you. When we experience traumatic stress, we try to avoid the memory to keep it from happening again. Read it out loud until it doesn't make you anxious anymore. At that point, whenever the memory comes around again, you will be capable of thinking of something good in your life. You can then go to the good. This process keeps you from avoiding the incident, which is called "cognitive restructuring." It is incredibly difficult to face, but by doing so, you can rewire your brain.

In conclusion, have hope! This is NOT an incurable disorder because there is relief available for you. Be confident to know that you, too, can overcome traumatic stress just like we have. Oscar Wilde once said, "Cages are not made of bars; they are made of our thoughts."

The past can turn on many irrational fear switches. Take a nightly inventory of all the positive things that happened to you during that day. Build your tomorrows on the positives of today.

PTSD is the past. Do not let it steal your present joy. We love you so much!

CHAPTER THIRTY-SIX
THE BEGINNING OF YOUR NEW BEGINNING

As you come to the end of this book, we close it the same way we began.

In a perfect world, you would have no problems.
In a perfect world, you would get along with everyone.
In a perfect world, you would weigh exactly what you wanted to weigh, have as much money as you want to have, and do everything you want to do.
In a perfect world, you would never have any challenges.
In a perfect world, there would be no stress.

We do not live in a perfect world. We live far, far from it. In the past, you may have felt like every day you were bombarded with this stress or that stress or old stress or new stress. If you are like the majority of people in the world, then you know what it is like to be stressed. The difference is, now you have permission to live your life stress-free.

Most people accept the fact that stress is best described as being in a situation you have no control over. You now have control.

While the creation of your new life will take time, patience, and multiple restarts, you now have the recipe you have been longing for to give yourself the lifestyle that you were designed to live.

We understand that there is no perfect world, and there is no such thing as an ideal life. There is just life. It will have countless ups and downs and twists and turns, but you can now handle it all. You can live well. It is our life's passion, our heart's desire, and our spiritual calling to provide you with every tool necessary to turn off your Stress Switches so that you can handle anything and everything that you experience in life.

A note from Matt:

My wife and I LOVE Christmas! We love everything about the season. Especially spending time with our friends and families. We also love doing whatever we can to spread the Christmas spirit and cheer to others.

On December 10, 2019, Katy and I had pulled out all the stops and were decorating our house and yard with all the festive trees, displays, and lights. Most of my time was spent outside putting lights on the house and the decorations in the yard. It was cold and windy outside, but I loved every minute of it. As the day drew to a close and we began to revel in the beauty of our décor, I noticed a few minutely small "dry weather" cracks on my hands – the apparent result of being outside in the dry, cold December air. Being accustomed to getting those throughout the winter months, I did not give them a second thought as we went to bed that night.

By 3:00 AM, I was awoken to a throbbing pain from one of the smallest cracks, located on the index finger of my left hand. The pain was quite intense, and I could feel every beat of my heart in that microscopic wound. I struggled to find any extra sleep for the rest of that night. When morning came, I applied more antibiotic cream on the wound and started to prepare for the day. Katy had to go to work, and I had to travel five hours to Albuquerque, NM, to conduct a leadership training seminar. Due to my lack of rest the night before, my mom had agreed to go with me, and I was incredibly grateful.

I rested as much as possible while she drove me to my speech. Afterward, we met my amazing cousin and his wife for dinner. While we were dining together, I felt chills begin to come over my body. I knew then that I had an infection that was going to require a doctor's help. After another restless night's sleep, the first thing the next morning, I scheduled an appointment at a local wellness clinic. I assumed that I would see a doctor, get some antibiotics, and then we could be on our way back home.

My appointment was for 11:30 AM. Before the appointment, mom and I had breakfast with my dear friend, who is the editor of this very book. During breakfast, she noticed that red streaks were beginning to make their way up my arm. We knew then that I was facing a much more serious situation. So, we headed to the wellness clinic. As soon as the doctor walked in the examination room and noticed the infection in my finger and the redness of my arm, she exclaimed, "OH (expletive)!!! YOU HAVE TO GET TO AN EMERGENCY ROOM NOW!" Talk about someone stressing you out!

She immediately made arrangements with the closest hospital, and within minutes of walking into the Emergency Room, they called me back. In short order, I was examined by three doctors, blood drawn, and they discovered a bacterial infection that had found its way into my body through a crack in my finger no larger than a paper cut. Intravenous antibiotics were started immediately.

To flush out the infected finger, a surgical procedure was scheduled for the next available opening in the operating room. Katy and her best friend got on the road as soon as we realized how serious the situation had become. After the surgery, the doctor informed us that had I waited another hour to get to the hospital, they would not have been able to save my finger. If I had waited another day to get to go to the Emergency Room, in his words, "The infection would have been in your bloodstream, and that would have been a REALLY bad day for you."

Three days later, I was released from the hospital and sent home with nine different prescriptions.

Unfortunately, after Christmas, the infection reared its ugly head again, leading to 10 days of the most potent oral antibiotics a person can take. The infection was cleared, but the lingering effects of swelling, stiffness, and pain remained. Because of the nerve damage from the infection and the aggressiveness of the procedure, the doctor said it could take up to one year before we know what the permanent effects are going to be.

As of the writing of this chapter, it has been two months. The entire situation is still so very surreal to me. The crack in my finger was TINY, yet somehow and from somewhere, an infection found the opening, which gave birth to multiple levels of significant stress.

I share that story with you now to hopefully impress upon you the importance of taking care of even the smallest of stresses, because even the seemingly insignificant can take root and cause incredible difficulties.

So many times, all of us can be guilty of focusing on the "major" stresses in life while we inadvertently turn away from hundreds of seemingly insignificant "minor" stress switches. Eventually, the minors accumulate one on the other and short circuit your ability to handle everyday life. Fortunately, you can now begin your journey of turning off those switches and turning on your new life.

The approach of Stress Free You is radically different from any other program you have ever heard of or seen. The tips and tricks that we have shared with you are groundbreaking, genuinely potent, occasionally controversial, and positively life-changing.

> **IF** you want to try again and succeed...
> **IF** you want to start again and win...
> **IF** you want to give it your all and wake up every morning with love, joy, peace, and a sound mind...

Then you deserve more than just stress relief; you deserve to live stress-free. We know you can do this!

Allow us to say again, “Welcome to Stress-Free You.”

CHAPTER THIRTY-SEVEN

THE ALPHABET OF STRESS EFFECTS

Angry people are not necessarily angry because they are angry.

Brusque people are not necessarily brusque because they are brusque.

Cranky people are not necessarily cranky because they are cranky.

Difficult people are not necessarily difficult because they are difficult.

Edgy people are not necessarily edgy because they are edgy.

Frustrated people are not necessarily frustrated because they are frustrated.

Gloomy people are not necessarily gloomy because they are gloomy.

Hard people are not hard because they are hard.

Ignorant people are just ignorant people.

Jerks are not necessarily jerks because they are jerks.

Kooky people are not necessarily kooky because they are kooky.

Lazy people are not necessarily lazy because they are lazy.

Mean people are not necessarily mean because they are mean.

Nasty people are not necessarily nasty because they are nasty.

Oppressive people are not necessarily oppressive because they are oppressive.

Panicky people are not panicky because they are panicky.

Quarrelsome people are not necessarily quarrelsome because they are quarrelsome.

Rude people are not necessarily rude because they are rude.

Self-absorbed people are not necessarily self-absorbed because they are self-absorbed.

Thoughtless people are not necessarily thoughtless because they are thoughtless.

Ungrateful people are not necessarily ungrateful because they are ungrateful.

Vengeful people are not necessarily vengeful because they are vengeful.

Weak people are not necessarily weak because they are weak.

Xenophobic people are not necessarily xenophobic because they are xenophobic.

Yucky people are not necessarily yucky because they are yucky.

Zany people are not necessarily zany because they are zany.

They are all people who may be very stressed!
And you are not one of them.

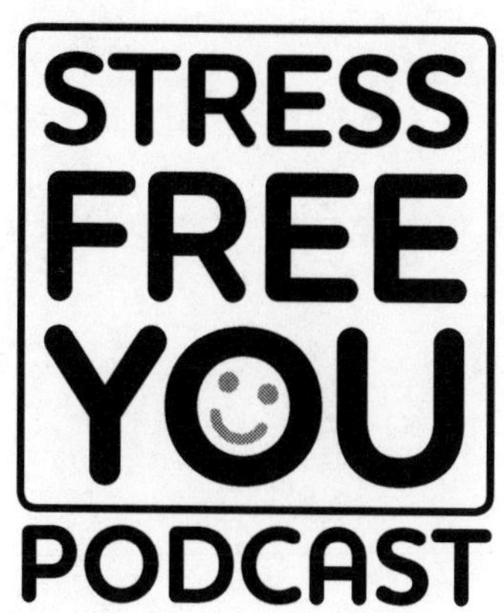

Imagine waking up each day with love, joy, peace, and a sound mind. Stress Free You is an innovative podcast about freeing yourself from the burden of stress so you can live a healthier, happier life. Rather than merely providing overly-simplistic tips, hosts Matt and Katy Rush and Rich Taylor examine stress from every angle, for a unique and more holistic approach. The three hosts methods for stress reduction are groundbreaking and occasionally controversial and stem from a desire to help others. Each episode opens with a skit about the day's topic, often just tongue-in-cheek enough to elicit a chuckle.

The Stress Free You podcast, available wherever you get your podcasts or visit: StressFreeYou.net/Podcast

Made in the USA
San Bernardino, CA
14 April 2020